BURSTING WITH ENERGY

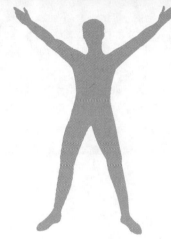

Optimum Energy And Permanent Weight Control At Any Age

Plus

A Breakthrough Test To Improve Your Energy Level, Biological Age, And Overall Health

By

Frank Shallenberger, M.D., H.M.D.

Medical Director,
The Nevada Center of Anti-Aging Medicine

Foreword By

Jonathan Wright, MD

NOTE TO THE READER

This book is not intended as medical advice or to replace medical care. It is meant exclusively for informational and educational purposes only, and not to diagnose, treat, or cure any disease. If you have symptoms or a disease, consult a qualified health professional. If you are currently taking prescription drugs, do not discontinue or substitute them for any suggestions described in this book without consulting your doctor.

As per federal guidelines, please be informed that the statements contained here have not been evaluated by the Food and Drug Administration.

Book design by Keith Gall/ Bajam Graphic Design, Los Angeles
Cover design by Lisa L. Cook/Blue Moon Advertising, Reno

Printed in the United States of America

Dedication

To my patients, the most wonderful group of people a doctor could ever hope to serve.

You have allowed me to "practice" on you for years.

You have given your trust and often bared your souls.

You have faced the uncertainty of sickness and the certainty of death with great strength and courage.

You have given me support when I needed it most, and have taught me more about life and medicine than all my medical books and training.

In you I have often been privileged to see the beauty and magnificence that humans are capable of. I feel humbled and honored in your presence.

This book is also dedicated to my wife and children, who have had to endure everything from coffee enemas to soy burgers as part of my particular search for truth.

Acknowledgments

Special thanks to Marty Zucker for his editorial guidance, great ideas, and professional writing skills. Without you Marty, this book would have been something close to a literary disaster. You have been an all-around pleasure to work with.

Also, thanks to Kathie Thompson, a great friend, a wonderful person, and a fabulous proof reader.

Table of Contents

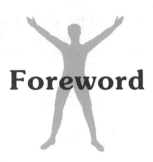

Foreword

Natural health care and natural medicine really aren't hard. We just need to "read our human blueprints" and follow them! It's just common sense. We do this if we're trying to maintain or repair anything else: Find the original plans, the original specifications, and work with or duplicate them. To repair broken equipment, we find parts identical to the damaged ones, put them in place just as the original plan specifies, and the equipment works again. No big deal. Maintenance is done like this all the time, everywhere.

Unless you're a doctor.

If you're a doctor, you try to repair humans with parts never, ever found in the original blueprints. Where the human biochemical plan calls for a protein or an amino acid, you use a patent medicine ("pharmaceutical drug"). Where the plan specifies a vitamin, you use a patent medicine. Where the plan calls for a combination of essential fatty acids, zinc, and vitamin A, you use….a patent medicine!

Is it any wonder that more than 100,000 of us in the USA reportedly die of "adverse reactions" to patent medicines? The real surprise is that patent medicines do any good at all, since they're simply not part of our original design.

It's as if an entire country's mechanics insisted on fixing automobiles with airplane parts! It wouldn't make any sense. Customers would be screaming at them to follow the original plan!

"Use automobile parts for automobiles, and never mind whether the Federal Automobile Administration 'approves' or not," the customers would demand. "It's just common sense!"

Dr. Frank Shallenberger is a very unusual doctor. He follows the "original human blueprint," even though he, too, was "educated" to use parts that have never, ever been part of the blueprint of human malfunction repair. And, for several years, he recommended patent medicines as he'd been taught in medical school. But after observing that "using airplane parts to fix automobiles" didn't work, he did something very unusual (for a doctor): He decided to figure out for himself what would really work, and in this book, he shares his discoveries with us.

Dr. Shallenberger went back to basic principles. He decided to apply the factors that have supported human life for literally hundreds of thousands of years (not one of them a patent medicine) and....they worked!

Water.

Rest.

Sunlight.

Food (*real* food, please!).

Exercise.

Breathing (healthfully).

Simple things, but things we all need to relearn in the 21st century (come to think of it, we humans have needed to re-learn them for several centuries!) since our "way of life" has departed so far from those of "original" humanity.

But Dr. Shallenberger doesn't expect or want us to live as original, primitive humans. He blends the factors that have helped keep humans healthy over thousands of generations with *real* improvements that modern scientific knowledge has brought to health care:

Supplements. (No one even *knew* about vitamins a century ago!).

Natural (not synthetic or horse) hormone replacement.

An advanced knowledge of human biochemistry that allows for much more accurate diagnosis and treatment.

And he's put together a testing system that (logically enough) measures your body's basic air intake and output to gauge how efficiently your body works. Even though his system is quite innovative, it's just common sense (again). It's just like testing automobile exhaust to determine how efficiently the engine works. Even better, if a malfunction is found, he can tell us how to fix it!

Please don't think that I'm unappreciative of some of the tremendous advances made in medicine over the last century. Dr. Shallenberger and I agree that if you get run over by a truck, it doesn't matter whether the truck carried whole, natural organic food or junk food. Either way, you will benefit greatly from skilled surgeons using the latest techniques guided by the most up-to-date diagnostic equipment. These areas of medicine are the best ever....it's just those patent medicines we have a big problem with!

The focus of this book isn't just health. It's health with plenty of energy to do whatever it is we want to do while we're here. And "bursting with energy" doesn't come from surgery or the latest diagnostic equipment. Energy comes from applying the basic principles taught in this book!

When I'm at a convention for natural medicine ("original human blueprint") doctors, I'm always happy and never disappointed when Dr. Shallenberger speaks to us. I always learn something from his insights.

I'm sure you will too!

Jonathan V. Wright, M.D.
Tahoma Clinic
Renton, Washington
www.tahoma-clinic.com

Author: *Why Stomach Acid is Good For You*
Maximize Your Vitality and Potency for Men Over 40
Natural Hormone Replacement for Women Over 45
(all written with Lane Lenard, Ph.D.)

Introduction
A Unifying Theory of Aging

There have been dozens of theories attempting to explain exactly what it is that causes the sickness and debility that we call aging. These include the free radical theory, the neuroendocrine theory, the damaged mitochondria theory, the Hayflick limit theory, the telemerase theory, and the "wear and tear" theory just to mention a few. For a good descriptive synopsis of all of the various theories of aging one can refer to *"Stopping the Clock"* (Keats Publishing), an excellent book on anti-aging medicine by Drs. Ronald Klatz and Robert Goldman.

Each of these theories has its own special attraction and logic, and each theory leads to its own particular therapeutic approach, which of course is designed to retard or reverse aging. **But a very significant problem with each and every one of these theories, especially to the patient and physician in the real world, is the fact that there is no good way to clinically judge whether the therapies stemming from any of these theories are actually working!**

For example, the free radical theory of aging states that aging is due to cellular damage from a class of molecules called free radicals, which are formed in the normal everyday course of metabolism. Therapies stemming from this theory focus on decreasing the amount of damage perpetrated by these molecules. But a major problem with the practical use of these anti-free radical treatments is that we don't have a practical way to assess if what we are doing is actually decreasing the rate of free radical damage.

Similarly, consider the case of the telemerase theory. Telemeres are molecules that are attached to the ends of our chromosomes, and they act to maintain the integrity of our DNA. Over time, with each division of our cells these telemeres become damaged, and according to the telemere theory of aging, it is the damaged telemeres that are primarily responsible for aging. All we have to do is to figure out some way to protect the telemeres from injury. Again, the biggest practical problem with using this theory is that there are no tests available to determine whether or not your anti-aging treatments are in fact doing that.

To give yet a third example, the neuroendocrine theory of aging states that aging results from the deterioration of hormone receptor activity in a part of the brain called the hypothalamus. It's a great theory, but so far we have no practical way of measuring hypothalamic receptor activity, and hence no way of knowing if our therapies are effective.

Unfortunately, the sobering truth is that each and every theory of aging is plagued with the curse that there is no good way to test or otherwise determine whether or not it actually has any therapeutic value in the real world.

That's problem number one, but another perhaps even more important problem with all these theories is that none of them offers the promise of one unifying theory that takes into account the rest of the other theories.

I am proposing an altogether different theory of aging, which I will call the energy deficit theory. This theory has the distinct advantage of being able to solve the two problems I just mentioned. Namely, there is an easy, inexpensive, and very practical way to actually measure whether or not anti-aging treatment strategies stemming from this theory are actually working. And secondly, it is a unifying theory.

The Energy Deficit Theory Of Aging

A paradigm is defined in the dictionary as a "clear and typical pattern." In practice it refers to a model or a way of thinking which best exemplifies the direction and inner workings of a given scientific system. For this reason, perhaps nothing is as important in any science as the paradigms it embraces.

Anti-aging medicine has its paradigms, many of which are a result of the various theories of aging mentioned above. Flowing forth from these paradigms is nothing less than the defined direction of all the endeavors directed at anti-aging therapy and research. In other words, the focus of anti-aging medicine is determined by its paradigms. This point is extremely important because one of the most basic assumptions among anti-aging medical paradigms is that the reduced energy production universally associated with aging is caused by the process of aging, i.e., **aging causes low energy production.**

My research, using a fascinating method called Bio-Energy Testing™ that measures the dynamics of my patients' energy production, has led me to a very radical departure from this assumption. Indeed, the results of my experience after testing and improving the energy production of hundreds of aged individuals have led me to formulate an entirely new paradigm, one that offers a unique perspective on aging and what can be done about it.

In short the new paradigm is this: **We don't decrease our energy production as a result of aging. Rather, we age as a result of decreased energy production, I.E., low energy production causes aging.** Or to put it another way, as long as an individual can maintain optimum energy production, that person will not age.

Let's look at some of the other theories of aging in view of this new paradigm:

The Free Radical Theory. It's not free radicals that result in aging and decreased energy production. It's decreased energy production that leads to free radical damage and aging.

The Telemere Theory. It's not that damaged telemeres result in aging and decreased energy production. It's decreased energy production that leads to damaged telemeres and aging.

The Neuroendocrine Theory. It's not the decreased hypothalamic receptor activity that leads to aging and decreased energy production. It's decreased energy production that causes decreased hypothalamic receptor activity resulting in aging.

In fact, every theory of aging so far advocated can be explained in terms of decreased energy production. Thus, one of the most compelling and attractive aspects of an energy deficit theory of aging is that it can explain all the phenomena that has led other investigators to arrive at each of the other theories of aging. This makes it a central, unifying theory of aging.

A Theory That Can Be Measured

But as a clinician who actually works everyday with real patients, by far the most exciting thing about this theory is that it can be tested and measured routinely in the clinic. In this way, such a theory has profound implications for measuring the efficacy of anti-aging strategies.

Instead of breaking down aging into its myriad symptoms and systems, one can simply ask one question: How can I increase my energy production to that of a younger person?

For example, if a particular herb is shown to increase my energy production, then according to this new paradigm, it will decrease my rate of aging. Similarly, if a particular practice such as meditation or sunbathing can increase energy production, then it will also retard the process of aging.

Using this new paradigm I have endeavored to discover what remedies and practices increase energy production, and in this way I believe that the door to unraveling the mysteries of the aging process, may be opened a little further

3

But...Is It Really Possible?

In June of 2000 I was invited to speak at The First International Learning Conference on Anti-Aging Medicine in Monte Carlo. My subject: How to set up an anti-aging clinic.

There was a fairly large contingency of physicians from China, where the government is interested in establishing a network of such clinics. During the question and answer session following my talk, one of the Chinese physicians asked me if I really thought it was possible to halt and even reverse the aging process.

My response was that it is not only possible, but that, in fact, I was already doing it in my clinic in Nevada.

I explained that the single best determinant of aging is the measurement of how efficiently an individual is able to produce energy. This capacity for energy production I refer to as the individual's Energy Quotient, or E.Q. for short, and it predictably and steadily declines with aging.

Using a testing technology I call Bio-Energy Testing™, I can now measure anyone's E.Q. quickly, easily, and with great precision. **With this method I have found that many of my 60 and 70-year-old patients, who follow the anti-aging guidelines you will be reading about in this book, are now producing energy as efficiently as a 40-year-old.** I believe that these people have literally stopped aging!

How Do You Want To Die?

Someone once said that as soon as you are born you start dying. This isn't quite true because we don't really start the dying part until somewhere around the age of 40, but the point is nonetheless well taken.

After age 40, unless we do something about it, our cells enter into a deterioration mode. With time, the rate of decline accelerates.

Have you ever asked yourself how and when you want to die? If you haven't, you should. **The reason is that if you want to live long and maintain your independence and function right up until the time you die, there are many things you must do (or stop doing, as the case may be), and the best time to take action is right now.** The younger the better.

Someday I will die, but until then I want to live a healthy and functional life. I don't want heart disease, diabetes, cancer, arthritis, dementia, or even the feebleness often considered an inevitable part of aging.

It is this strong desire that has compelled me through my professional life to discover as much as I could about the aging process, and how to slow it down. I now know that to a very large extent - barring an accident or some act of violence, of course - we are able to determine not only how and when we will die, but also more importantly how long and how well we will live.

My Story

I've been practicing medicine for almost thirty years, the last twenty of which have been devoted to researching and developing alternative medical strategies to increase the length and quality of my patients' lives.

Frequently, patients ask why I decided to pursue alternative medicine. It's a good question, especially since when I first began to investigate this field there was a stigma attached to it. The medical establishment regarded it as synonymous with quackery. The terms "complementary" and "alternative" had not been coined yet.

Times have certainly changed! Now there is an Office of Alternative Medicine at the National Institutes of Health. Hundreds of books have been written, and even the Journal of the American Medical Association, a leading voice of mainstream medicine, has dedicated whole issues to the subject. Many states have even passed legislation protecting doctors using natural medicine from unscrupulous persecution by medical licensing boards. But the climate was totally different, and actually hostile, back in the late seventies when I first became enamored with the idea of working with natural remedies to treat and prevent disease.

Symptoms Improved...But Not Patients

After I graduated from medical school in 1973, I received training in surgery and specialized in emergency medicine. I worked in this very exciting field for the next five years and then decided I needed a change.

I chose to open a general medicine practice across the street from the hospital emergency room where I had previously worked. I naively hung up my shingle and prepared to begin a new medical career. But did I ever have some lessons to learn.

Within six months I began to make the rather unsettling observation that none of my patients with chronic diseases were getting well. The ones with acute disorders - colds, flu, broken legs, cuts, and sprains - all got well, often regardless of my treatments.

But the patients with chronic conditions such as arthritis, diabetes, and heart disease, never showed any real improvement at all. Of course I was able to help their symptoms with drugs and surgery. They would feel better. Their medical tests would improve. Yet the same disease was still present.

Not only that, but many of them developed serious side effects and secondary medical conditions from the very treatments I was giving them.

Years later statistics would become available showing that more than 100,000 patients die annually as a result of *properly* administered medical therapy.

But back then I was just barely beginning to appreciate the depth of this problem.

My years in the emergency room had made me completely naive about how day-to-day medicine was practiced on patients with chronic conditions. In the emergency room, if a patient was brought in with a knife protruding from his head (as actually happened once), we didn't just give him some medication for the symptoms and send him home. We removed the knife, repaired the injuries, and then sent him home.

When a desperate patient reported that he could not breathe, we tried to quickly determine the cause, and then go about to remedy it. We didn't just send him home with oxygen.

In emergency medicine you directly treat the cause of the problem, not just the symptoms. I had become so used to asking why patients have the symptoms they have that I just assumed that practitioners of chronic medicine did that as well. But I was in for a big surprise.

A few months after I launched my general medicine practice, one of my arthritic patients developed an ulcer, the result of taking a standard medication that I had prescribed. The incident alarmed me greatly. I felt I had failed the patient.

I decided to discuss the situation with some of the best physicians in the community at the time. I compared notes on how they treated various diseases and how I treated the same conditions. I learned that I was pretty much following the conventional wisdom.

"...We Can't Treat Causes..."

I then received from one of those doctors a life-changing piece of information. I held this particular doctor in great esteem. What he told me was this: "Frank, you're doing just fine. When it comes to the treatment of chronic diseases, you have to accept the fact that at this point in time we can't treat causes, because nobody knows what the causes are. The best we can do is simply to make our patients feel better, and try to avoid complications with the intelligent and judicious use of medication."

Could it be, I thought, that the reason nobody knows what causes disease is because nobody is asking the question?

This started me wondering just what kinds of things could possibly serve as the cause or causes of chronic diseases. In medical school we looked at the results of disease: the pathology. But no time was spent on the possible causes of disease.

It was around this time that I happened to pull out an old publication on vitamins that my dad had received from a drug company back in the early fifties. I started to read it and found myself devouring the information. I recall looking under the symptoms of deficiencies of different vitamins and seeing arthritis, diabetes, rashes, colitis, hypothyroidism, cancer, heart disease, anxiety, depression, and virtually every other chronic illness for which "there is no known cause." In the one whole hour my medical school dedicated to nutrition we were taught that these kinds of deficiencies only occurred in serious starvation situations, and certainly not among average Americans.

I now began to wonder about that assumption.

The Linus Pauling Approach

In the summer of 1980, I learned about a conference on "Orthomolecular Medicine" in San Francisco. The conference was organized by physicians who had been influenced by two-time Nobel Prize winner Linus Pauling, Ph.D. Pauling believed that diseases were caused by delicate imbalances in the body's biochemistry, and that these diseases could be prevented and often reversed simply by correcting these imbalances. He called the concept "orthomolecular" because it involved restoring the right ("ortho") molecule to the body at the right time.

I anxiously went to the conference hoping to gain insight into the questions I had been pondering. I was not disappointed.

I heard about reversing and even curing heart disease, hypertension, gout, arthritis, headaches, anxiety, and schizophrenia merely through the scientific use of vitamins and minerals. Better yet, I learned how many of these conditions could be prevented using the same concepts.

I heard from medical pioneers who had been successfully using these treatments for years. I was most happy to hear that none of these doctors made their patients worse by creating other disorders from the side effects of pharmaceuticals.

While the rest of medicine was busy pursuing the use of treatments that routinely caused death and injury from side effects, these physicians looked for safe and effective alternatives. **Although at the time I hadn't been sure of where I was going in my medical career, I knew then and there that I wanted to go wherever these doctors were headed.**

Back then, except for an occasional conference like this, there was no place to learn how to proceed. There were very few books available.

So I developed a set of criteria for the application of "unproven," alternative techniques. First, I reasoned, they must be inherently safe. Secondly, they must either have a good anecdotal record or be theoretically reasonable. Lastly, they must be inexpensive.

Using these criteria as my guide, I began to take myself and my patients down an exciting and rewarding path.

Two decades later, I can honestly say that I made the right decision to follow this path. I have been able to help thousands of patients in ways that I couldn't possibly have done with my conventional medical education.

Many alternative treatments really correct the causes of disease. Many diseases still considered incurable are, in fact, curable and for the most part, easily preventable. Even aging itself is very treatable.

But patients need to find doctors who use these methods. Unfortunately, the medical establishment is still controlled by the pharmaceutical industry. And the side effects of their products kill more than 100,000 people a year, with another 1 million injured so severely that they require hospitalization.

This book was written to help you avoid being part of those statistics.

The Golden Years?

A patient once told me that the "golden years" were the years when you needed more gold to pay for special medical attention, medications, or nursing homes. You were unemployed and virtually condemned to live on the dole.

Indeed, this concept of what it's like to get old is so common that when I first began to discuss the idea of living longer, many patients were rather dismissive.

"I'll deal with that later," they would say. "Why bother myself with that while I am still feeling well? I want to focus on the positive, and besides, no one wants to live forever."

True, no one wants to live forever, but all of us would like to live our "golden years" free from the diseases and frailties that so commonly characterize this period. And free from constant doctors' visits, multiple medications, and nursing homes. And free to feel young, to be employed, to go fishing with our great grandchildren, to hike up the mountain, to have sex, to maybe go back to school, or just free to really enjoy another beautiful day.

It seems that Nature really plays a dirty trick on all of us, because it weakens and deteriorates us just when we have gained the wisdom and experience to really appreciate the beauty that life has to offer. Just when we realize that being alive and feeling strong is a blessing, we are rudely interrupted by a damaged heart and the need for someone to drive us to the cardiologist.

Me, 100 Years Old!?

They say you could live to be more than a hundred years old. And they're right. According to the World Health Organization, "there have been more gains in life expectancy in the last fifty years than in the previous five thousand years."

The U.S. Census Bureau has gone on record to say that "by the year 2025 there will be two 65-year-olds for every teenager in America."

So the odds are looking better and better that you will live to be quite old. The question then becomes, what do you want it to be like, and what can you do about it.

Recent advances in medical research have led to the growing realization that much of the mental and physical decline traditionally perceived as an inevitable consequence of aging can, in fact, be delayed, prevented, and often even reversed. Indeed, medical science is finally learning that aging, and all of the symptoms that go with it, is a treatable condition.

As you will see from reading this book, diseases associated with aging are already preventable. So, too, is the functional decline in mental and physical ability.

The suffering and disability that we have been so used to seeing in the elderly does not have to be a part of our lives.

And perhaps the best news is that achieving these benefits is becoming easier. Moreover, you don't have to be rich to make the golden years really golden.

The Future Is Here, Now

Anti-aging research has demonstrated that the human equivalent of living a fully functional life for a hundred and fifty years can be achieved in animals.

The new medical specialty of anti-aging medicine is now spurring on this research and making it an increasing reality for humans.

Anti-aging medicine is the medicine of the future and you are the patient of the future. The day is coming when the thought of waiting until you are sick to see the doctor will be as silly and archaic as not cleaning your hands before surgery. In this new medicine, patients are seeking medical advice, and are being placed on aggressive health enhancing and disease prevention programs while they are still young and healthy **before** they develop disease.

The American Academy of Anti-Aging Medicine was formed in 1993 in response to the growing interest among physicians and researchers. There are now hundreds of physicians all over the world who are board-certified specialists in Anti-Aging Medicine.

Ronald Klatz, M.D., president of the organization, predicted in 1999 that a full "50 percent of all baby boomers alive and well today will celebrate their 100th birthday with physical and mental faculties intact." The question is will you be among them, and what will your life be like if your are?

Part One
You Are Your Energy Level

Chapter 1
Energy Production:
The Real Generation Gap

Harry, Before

Five years ago, Harry, at age 77, went to his doctor complaining of insomnia, fatigue, lack of stamina, weakness, stiff, achy joints and muscles, and a decreased interest and enjoyment in life.

His doctor ran the usual battery of tests, and told Harry the one thing he really didn't want to hear: "You are perfectly healthy for your age."

Harry knew better. He knew that "perfectly healthy" did not describe him. He left the doctor's office feeling depressed. If this was what it was like to feel "perfectly healthy" for his age now, what did the future bode?

Harry was a man of action, and always had been. He wanted more out of life, no matter how old he was. Drawing on an inherently resilient nature, he shoved aside the depression, discarded the doctor's verdict, and set out to recharge his battery.

Harry, After

Today, Harry is 82. He exercises daily. He has 18 percent body fat and good musculature. His mental function tests reveal a fully functional brain with scores almost as good as those of a 22-year-old.

His energy production is more like someone thirty years younger than someone his age. He sleeps well, with an average of eight hours of good sleep per night. He wakes up feeling fresh and full of vigor.

He still backpacks up the same trails that he trekked more than half a century ago. His balance is good. He roller skates, cycles, and skis with ease.

His mood is exceptional. He has passion for life, and is always keen to engage and solve new problems.

He has full sexual function.

His muscles and joints are flexible and free of the pains and stiffness that so many of his contemporaries suffer.

In short, Harry feels and functions at an optimum level.

Caroline, Before

Caroline had just passed her 46th birthday when she came to see me. She was in bad shape.

For the previous five years she had been plagued with fatigue, insomnia, menstrual disorders, depression, and all sorts of aches and pains. She had gained thirty pounds for no apparent reason, and couldn't lose weight even with exercise and a good diet.

She had seen several different specialists who diagnosed her variously with chronic fatigue syndrome, fibromyalgia, hypothyroidism, and depression. More than once she had been told to remember that she was "not getting any younger," and that "for her age" she wasn't really doing all that bad.

Caroline had different symptoms than Harry, but the doctors were giving her the same age-related nonsense.

Caroline's doctors prescribed sleeping pills, pain pills, and antidepressants, but never gave her any hope for curing or reversing her problems. Indeed, they didn't seem to really know just what her problems were.

Like Harry, she also found herself depressed by her medical treatments. What kind of future did she have if she was already feeling this bad before turning fifty?

Caroline, After

When I first tested Caroline, her energy production was equivalent to that of a 92-year- old!

"No wonder I feel like an old lady," she lamented. "From all functional aspects, I am!"

That was then.

But today, Caroline, like Harry, has remade herself.

After we confirmed her low energy status using a remarkable new testing technology called Bio-Energy Testing™, we pinpointed the problems causing it, and designed a remedial program to correct them. There were many problems: a deficiency of thyroid and adrenal hormones, along with poor fitness, too much stress, and improper breathing.

Caroline lacked the energy to fight off an ordinarily benign virus called the Epstein-Barr virus, or EBV for short. This bug is often cited as the culprit in chronic fatigue states. Her previous physicians had focused on eradicating the virus rather than on her real problem: an energy deficit that weakened her immune system.

Caroline's thyroid level was low, but was not addressed by her doctors because they relied on conventional blood testing, which is often inaccurate, and her test results were still within the normal range.

Her symptoms caused her much stress and led to an adrenal insufficiency that was never tested and thus overlooked.

Within six weeks of instituting a program that treated all these abnormalities, her energy testing already showed improvement.

In another three months she was starting to feel energetic for the first time in many years.

Within another six months Caroline had lost thirty pounds and was back to working full time. Her energy production was now that of a 43-year-old, and she had developed an entirely fresh and enthusiastic attitude toward life.

"Age Related Symptoms"

Before she remade herself, Caroline was a relatively young person with the energy level of a much older person.

And Harry, after he remade himself, was an older person with the energy production of a much younger individual.

Certainly these are dramatic cases, however, many of you may be able to identify to some degree with their so-called "age related symptoms."

Harry and Caroline's symptoms are collectively known as age related because they result solely from the aging process itself. **In other words, age related symptoms are not caused by a disease or psychological condition.**

Another way of putting it is that you can have all of these symptoms and be considered "perfectly healthy" for your age.

Common age related symptoms include the following:

❑   Vision and hearing impairment

❑   Anxiety and depression

❑   Insomnia

❑   Weakness, fatigue, and decreased stamina

❑   Weight gain and increased body fat

- ❑ Decreased sexual desire and function
- ❑ Dry, loose, wrinkled skin, and age spots
- ❑ Decreased memory, mental speed, and clarity
- ❑ Decreased balance
- ❑ Decreased energy
- ❑ Increased joint and muscle pain
- ❑ High cholesterol

For most of us the aging process begins around thirty-five, though it may be five or ten years later before noticeable symptoms occur. For some it begins earlier; for others much later.

Lifestyle factors, such as diet, smoking, and exercise, play a significant influence as to when symptoms show up.

Just remember this: long before we actually see the first signs of aging, the process has already been gong on, and age related symptoms are on the way. It's not a case of "if," it's a case of "when."

What's Your E.Q.?

In my opinion, Caroline, Harry, and every other case of "age related symptoms," no matter what the age, all have something in common. **That common something is decreased energy production stemming from a loss in the efficiency in which the body produces energy from oxygen.**

I call it a low E.Q. A low Energy Quotient. And a low E.Q. represents a real energy crisis.

If you'd like a very dramatic insight into the effects of a low E.Q., just hold your breath while reading the next few sentences.

Of course, decreased energy production from a decreased E.Q. is not quite so drastic as holding your breath. Indeed it is often very subtle. Sometimes patients are even able to exercise "as good as ever" without complaining about shortness of breath.

If their blood and tissue oxygen levels are tested, the results almost always fit well within acceptable limits, and yet their cells may be starving for the basic energy requirements that can only be met by an optimal E.Q.

To understand how this can occur, we need first to learn how the body uses oxygen to make energy, and what happens when this process is insufficient, even subtly.

And we need also to learn how to optimize the process when it is insufficient.

This book will give you these vital instructions.

Live Old - Die Young

The consideration of decreased energy production as a cause of aging is largely overlooked in modern medical practice, even geriatrics, where the predominant emphasis is simply on treatment of symptoms. It is primarily only among physicians like myself, who are interested in anti-aging concepts, where you will find any recognition and application of this concept.

Twenty-five years ago, when I first became interested in anti-aging medicine, nobody had much of a clue about this at all. I vividly remember my dad, who is an excellent physician with over half a century experience telling me: "Your patients are going to die anyway. The only thing that you are going to accomplish is that they are going to die in better shape."

"That's precisely the point," I replied.

Of course many of us in the anti-aging field are interested in increasing the length of our lives, but we should never lose sight of the greater good, that is, it is much more important to live *well* than to live *long*.

I personally hope to do both. I envision myself passing away in "great shape," free in large part from the incapacity, limitations, and diseases that so frequently affect the elderly. The key to accomplishing this is through optimizing my energy production to the level of a younger man.

What This Book Can Do For You

The purpose of this book is to help you do that as well.

If you are presently healthy, vigorous, and operating on all cylinders, you've probably got a pretty good E.Q. You're bursting with energy. And the information on these pages can help you function even better and keep you at that optimum level for all the years to come.

If you are less than vigorous and energetic, suffer from ill health, or are over the age of fifty you've got a sub-optimal E.Q. You're bursting all right, but without energy. The information here can help you bring up your energy quotient and enhance the body's self-healing mechanisms.

In either case, the information can boost energy production and slow down your rate of aging.

17

You won't find any of this information in another book, or in the medical library. It is based on years of working with patients and learning the "secrets" that improve their energy production, vigor, and health...at all ages.

Using a new testing technology called Bio-Energy Testing™, I've been able to establish optimum values related to your metabolism, Energy Quotient, fat burning ability, and other key markers that can help you hone in on optimal energy production. With this method I have been able to quantify and confirm the effects of these age defying "secrets."

I'll share these target values with you in Part One of the book, so that if you wish to pursue the path of high energy you will have a set of physiological references for it. I'll also explain the basics of how your body produces energy and how this process can go wrong. I'll explain as well how Bio-Energy Testing™ can help you correct and optimize your E.Q. so that you'll be "bursting with energy" for a long, long time.

Then, in Part Two, I will sequentially unfold the clinical "secrets" with you. There are ten of them. They involve lifestyle changes, some very simple, and some involving a bit of effort on your part, but all hugely rewarding. These "secrets" have the potential to raise your energy to a level you may have experienced only in your younger days, or in many cases, to a height you never imagined possible for you.

The younger you are when you first start making the changes and the longer you stay with them, the more effectively they will work for you. I tell patients not to wait until they are dragging before they get into an anti-aging program. Sure, it will help you even if you start late in life, but to enjoy an optimum energy level longer, I advise starting this kind of a program earlier on.

Feeling young is a lifetime endeavor. Make it habitual, and you will live longer and more importantly enjoy your life more.

As you read through the information you will note how the various components work together in a classic holistic sense. In other words, how you eat affects how you exercise, how you exercise affects how you sleep, how you sleep affects how you view life, how you view life affects how you eat and exercise.

For this reason, I would like you to regard the individual "secrets" in this book as threads in a fabric. You are the weaver. You take the threads. You put them together and they produce a beautiful fabric. Incorporate them comfortably into your life in stages, but make sure your goal is to eventually include *all* of them.

So don't feel overwhelmed and think you need to adopt them all at once. You will be pleased to observe, as I guide you through one, and then another, that your energy level is getting better and better.

And you'll be hooked.

Energy can be very addictive, you see.

If you follow the guidelines, I promise you'll become an energy addict. And making you one, and making you healthier and more youthful in the process, is why I have written this book.

Chapter 2
How Your Body Makes Energy

The Aerobic Process

Your body produces energy two ways: aerobically and anaerobically. Aerobic production refers to energy that comes from oxygen, while anaerobic production is created without oxygen. The two mechanisms are totally different. Let's take a moment and see how they work.

First aerobic, because that's the most important process.

Inside the trillions of cells in our body, molecules of oxygen, hydrogen, sugar, fat, vitamins, minerals, and amino acids pass through an assembly line of enzymatic processing that generates an enormous amount of energy. About 60 percent of this energy is used to produce heat. The remaining 40 percent is used to fuel every single physiological and biochemical reaction in the body.

A fairly reliable way to determine your aerobic energy production is to gauge how easily you become chilled or if your body temperature is below normal.

Yet another indicator of low aerobic energy production is the most frequent complaint from patients heard by doctors: "I feel tired."

In reality, poor aerobic energy production causes a decrease in energy that results in much more than simply being tired and cold. **More than any other single factor, it is the cause of aging and the diseases associated with aging.**

As I mentioned before, I have coined the term E.Q. (Energy Quotient) to refer to your ability to produce energy aerobically. Just like with your I.Q., the higher your E.Q. is, the better off you are.

Remember when you could easily bounce up three or four flights of stairs? Now you get winded after even one flight. That's because your E.Q. has decreased.

As you age, your E.Q. steadily falls in a linear fashion, and this decline is a solid indicator of your functional or "biological" age.

Your E.Q. can now be precisely measured using Bio-Energy Testing™. I will explain this exciting method in detail in the following chapter. It offers the most complete and exact measurement of health and aging that I have ever encountered in all my years of practicing preventive and anti-aging medicine.

This diagnostic tool gives you a practical yardstick on your current E.Q., and therefore, your current energy status. Then, at a later date, after you take action to improve your E.Q., you can retest yourself and see just how well you are progressing.

And here's the key point: anything that improves your E.Q. makes you functionally younger.

The Anaerobic Process

Anaerobic metabolism is a way for the cells to get extra energy without using oxygen. Nature designed it for emergencies, such as when trying to escape from a lion that has you in its sight for a next meal. The process kicks in when a very high amount of energy is needed for a very short period of time. Anaerobic energy production normally occurs on a limited basis as an everyday part of cellular function. This is considered completely normal and healthy.

When aerobic energy production is decreased as measured by a low E.Q., anaerobic production is increased to make up for the deficit. **It is this increased level of anaerobic energy production that accounts for many of the aches and pains and other common infirmities of aging.**

A common reason for the development of a low E.Q. and the subsequent increase in anaerobic energy production is a decreased delivery of oxygen to the tissues. Another is a dysfunction of the energy producing structures inside cells called the mitochondria. **Both of these situations are discussed later in this book, and routinely occur as a result of the following: dehydration, sunlight deficiency, poor nutrition, inadequate sleep, excessive dietary carbohydrate, deficient dietary protein, poor fitness, improper breathing, and hormonal deficiencies.**

Here's why the anaerobic process is so much less desirable than the aerobic process:

❑ It generates only a fraction of the energy produced by the aerobic process.

❑ It generates a high level of free radicals, highly destructive molecular fragments that damage DNA and cell membranes. They are considered a major cause of accelerated aging.

❑ It also creates high levels of lactic acid, a waste product that causes breathlessness and burning pain in your muscles when you exercise hard. As you age, you begin to increasingly experi ence these symptoms with a less intense level of exertion. The body is simply losing its ability to produce energy aerobically, and is forced to rely more on anaerobic production. **Thus, the entire process of energy production becomes compro- mised, your E.Q. slips, and you start to see and feel the effects of aging.**

Decreased E.Q. = Increased Aging and Disease

Whether it is a brain cell sparking a thought or a parietal cell initiating your digestion, every aspect of your physiology is 100 percent depen- dent on aerobic energy production. Your liver crucially depends on it. Your hair and skin. Your sex organs. Your vision. Your strength. Every- thing.

Nothing is nearly as important to your health and to your experience of life as the energy you produce from oxygen.

Without aerobic energy production you can't think, move, reproduce, resist infection, detoxify yourself, or make a structural protein or an enzyme.

You can't do anything!

And overwhelmingly, *every* clinical disorder that humans develop as they age is associated with an *insufficient E.Q.*

This is why I have spent the last seven years researching how to both *measure* and *improve* E.Q. What I have learned through research, clinical experience, and feedback from patients, I am now passing on to you.

Ever wonder why young people rarely develop disease despite their typical excesses, a high level of stress, lack of sleep, the worst of diets, and smoking? How do they manage to stay out all night long and come back for more activity the next day? The answer ultimately lies in their incredible E.Q.

By understanding the factors involved in how our bodies use oxygen to make energy, I believe it is possible not only to prevent all the dis- eases associated with getting older, but also to significantly slow down the very process of aging itself.

The Oxygen Odyssey

It all starts with the air we breath. Human beings, and indeed all living creatures, inhale the oxygen present in the air, extract and process it in the body, and exhale carbon dioxide. If it were not for the plant kingdom, we would have become extinct long ago, having used up all the oxygen available on the planet.

Fortunately, Nature blessed us with plants that are able to use the sun's energy to convert the carbon dioxide that we produce back into the oxygen that we so desperately need.

So next time you see the sun or a tree be sure to offer a prayer of thanks. *All life on earth depends on them!*

Depending on where you live, the air you breath contains from 20-23 percent oxygen. If you live in a metropolitan area or at a high altitude, the oxygen content will be less. If you live at sea level or in a rural area with lots of trees and vegetation, oxygen will be more abundant.

No matter where you live, however, your body adapts to the level of ambient oxygen.

❑ Step 1 Your Lungs

The first step in the utilization of oxygen is taking in a breath. This draws oxygen into the lungs where it can be picked up by the blood.

In this process, oxygen atoms bind to iron atoms in hemoglobin, protein molecules present in red blood cells. The oxygen is transported by the hemoglobin and delivered to the cells throughout the body.

The more hemoglobin you have, the more oxygen you can take up.

Cigarette smoke and other forms of atmospheric pollution bind up a percentage of the hemoglobin and interfere with its ability to take up and carry oxygen. In fact, exposure to just one cigarette worth of smoke significantly reduces the oxygen carrying capability of the blood for about 48 hours.

Diseases of the lungs such as asthma, bronchitis, and emphysema also decrease the blood's ability to transport oxygen.

Improper breathing is an even more common cause of interference with oxygen uptake. Later on I will discuss the importance of breathing correctly and offer some guidelines on how to adopt a more healthy breathing "style."

But assuming that you don't have a lung disease, and you don't smoke or live or work in a contaminated environment, and that you breathe correctly, you will be able to saturate your hemoglobin with oxygen. This is the first step to assuring an optimal E.Q.

❑ Step 2 Your Heart and Circulation

Your oxygen saturated blood then travels to the heart, which works non-stop to pump it throughout your body.

Did you know that the more you exercise the stronger the ability of your heart to pump blood? A heart that pumps optimally helps you meet all your energy needs by sending your oxygen saturated blood out to the trillions of cells, and then returning it to the lungs to pick up another load of oxygen.

The heart functions better when its stroke volume (the amount of blood carried with each beat) is optimal, and when it is capable of beating fast enough. Both stroke volume and maximum heart rate decline with aging and with decreased fitness. Conversely, they improve with anti-aging therapy and fitness programs.

❑ Step 3 Your Arteries

The heart is half the equation in this delivery system. Your arteries are the other half. It is through the arterial system that blood is carried to the tissues and cells from the heart.

As I mentioned, your heart is a pump. However, unlike a centrifugal pump with a constant output, the heart pumps in beats.

For maximum efficiency, the arteries need to be flexible, so that when the heart pushes out a volume of blood, the arteries can expand to accommodate the sudden increase in pressure. Then, when the heart relaxes between beats, the arteries must contract back to their original shape in preparation for the next beat.

This flexibility of the arteries is just as important to an adequate circulation as the heart itself. When arteries lose flexibility, and become constricted, due to stress, aging, and other factors, the frequent result is an elevation of blood pressure. High blood pressure or hypertension, are the medical terms used.

Although blood pressure readings are a good indicator, today we have more sensitive ways to measure the loss of arterial flexibility, which use transducers that can measure micro changes in arterial elasticity. We often discover loss of arterial flexibility even in persons with normal blood pressure readings. The degree to which your blood pressure becomes elevated above what it was in your younger years, even though the readings may still be in a so-called "acceptable range," reflects the degree to which your arteries have lost their flexibility and hence compromised your circulation.

Compromised circulation means decreased oxygen delivery. People with a poorly conditioned heart often have significant arterial stiffness with a "normal" resting blood pressure because their heart stroke volume is so low. In these cases their blood pressure will not become elevated until they begin to exercise.

When deposits of plaque develop on arterial walls, one is said to have a condition called atherosclerosis. This results in a hardening and narrowing of the arteries, further choking oxygen delivery. When this condition becomes advanced it can set the stage for deadly heart attacks or strokes.

❑ Step 4 Your 2,3 DPG Level

Your oxygenated blood is now coursing through many thousands of miles of arteries, arterioles (smaller arteries) and tiny capillaries. Now, it takes a special enzyme called 2,3 DPG to cut the bond between the hemoglobin and oxygen so that the oxygen can be released to the cells.

Without enough of this enzyme present, the hemoglobin, riding aboard the red blood cells, would simply cruise right on through without giving up the oxygen.

People who don't regularly exercise, or who have elevated insulin levels, or who have diabetes, have decreased levels of 2,3 DPG. They are unable to adequately utilize oxygen even in the presence of the normal functioning of lungs, heart, and arteries. Their blood oxygen levels may be quite normal, but this is very misleading because the oxygen can't get to the cells. And when oxygen can't get to the cells you might as well be holding your breath.

❑ Step 5 Your Mitochondria

The addresses for oxygen delivery in your body are the mitochondria located inside each cell. These microscopic structures are the power plants of the cells. Inside of them, special enzymes process oxygen, fats, and carbohydrates. Out of this complex process comes energy to drive the functions of the particular cell, along with water and carbon dioxide as by-products.

The mitochondria are very complex structures influenced by diet, toxicity, genetics, and hormones. As we age, these cellular dynamos become especially vulnerable to damage.

Many anti-aging experts believe that damaged mitochondria may, in fact, be responsible for virtually all of the diseases and infirmities of aging. For sure, poorly functioning mitochondria can drastically decrease your energy production, causing you to age much more rapidly.

Because of the incredible importance of optimal mitochondrial function to our health, I want to now focus at this point on how your mitochondrial function can be sabotaged.

How Your Mitochondria Are Undermined

As I mentioned a moment ago, it is inside the mitochondria of trillions of cells where the energy is produced to keep you thinking and moving.

Adequate oxygen delivery to the mitochondria is fundamental to this process. Thus, sedentary, unfit people are not assisting their mitochondria to do their job. No wonder they commonly complain of poor energy.

But there are plenty of other ways that mitochondrial function is undermined. And by correcting these problems you can restore your mitochondria back to more efficient - and youthful - function.

This is a huge issue. Of all the ways that energy production is impaired, poorly functioning mitochondria is the most significant and most common. In addition, it is the one cause that is almost always missed by conventional medical diagnosis. Bio-Energy Testing™ is unique because it can determine mitochondrial function. I'll talk about this revolutionary technology in a following chapter.

❑ **Hormonal Deficiency**

The inner intelligence regulating your body, namely in the form of hormones, determines how much energy your cells produce. If the body needs increased energy, certain hormones turn on cellular energy production in much the same way that a light switch turns on the light. If there is a deficiency in these messenger biochemicals - such as thyroid hormone, human growth hormone, progesterone, cortisol, and testosterone - the cells may not get "turned on." The degree to which these hormones are deficient actually determines your E.Q. more than anything else...and hence how well you age.

❑ **Mitochondrial Damage**

If the mitochondria become damaged, the energy process suffers.

Short-term exposure to harmful chemicals such as pesticides can cause damage. More commonly, there's a long-term impact from the so-called "heavy metals" - mercury, arsenic, lead, and cadmium - that slowly build up over the years inside the body.

Not only has elevated levels of mercury crept into tuna and other fish, but the mercury contained in silver dental fillings, has been shown to "leak" into the body and have a detrimental effect.

Additionally, lead, arsenic, and cadmium have become ubiquitous in our food and water supply. Well water or tap water from the faucets of high rises and old buildings can frequently be problematic. Even if a current water supply is clean, individuals may have accumulated toxic levels as a result of previously drinking contaminated water.

Heavy metals are insidious. They accumulate slowly in the body over many years. Moreover, the organs of elimination do not readily remove them. Earlier exposure to heavy metals will thus be present in the body many years later. I have often seen middle-aged patients with a decreased energy quotient secondary to mitochondrial damage sustained from playing with mercury, or quicksilver as it is also known, as far back as their childhood.

This chronic form of toxicity from heavy metals is often difficult to determine. A poor E.Q. may be the only telltale sign.

Other common causes of mitochondrial damage include viral and free radical injury to RNA and DNA.

❏ Adrenal Insufficiency From Stress

The main reason why mitochondria in the brain (and to a lesser extent in the rest of the body) don't function well is because of a shortage of glucose (sugar). Deficient glucose occurs as the result of a condition known as low blood sugar or hypoglycemia, present to one degree or another in every patient with any illness. It often occurs even in healthy people

Every cell in the body has the ability to create energy from either glucose or fat - every cell except brain cells. The brain can only utilize glucose. Therefore low blood glucose affects the brain far more than it does other organ systems.

Low blood sugar is by far the most common cause of brain dysfunction symptoms such as low energy, headaches, insomnia, poor mental clarity and concentration, anxiety, depression, moodiness, ADD, and hyperactivity. Unfortunately, conventional physicians often miss this diagnosis.

Low blood sugar results from chronic stress and excessive carbohydrate consumption.

Let's take stress first.

Stress comes in many forms: mental and emotional fatigue, allergies, injuries, pain, exposure to toxins, illness, infections, drugs and pharmaceuticals, inadequate rest, dehydration, nutrient deficiencies, and sunlight deficiency.

The body is well equipped to deal with stress, thanks in particular to the adrenal glands. These tiny glands, located just above the kidneys, produce many hormones. Among other things, these hormones help put the body back into balance after exposure to stress.

As long as stresses aren't too severe or don't last too long, the adrenals can do their jobs. **However, too much stress eventually results in fatigued and exhausted glands unable to produce an adequate amount of hormones**. Since a primary function of the adrenal glands is to maintain a healthy blood sugar level, the end result of chronically overworked adrenals is low blood sugar.

The late Hans Selye, M.D., who pioneered the understanding of how stress contributes to disease, confirmed in experiments how prolonged stress gradually wears out the adrenal glands. When this happens, the mitochondria in the brain cells become deprived of their only source of energy, and all the symptoms of low blood glucose emerge.

Unfortunately, many of the remedies used to counteract symptoms of low blood glucose involve substances such as coffee, alcohol, and medications. They only serve to weaken the adrenals even more!

As long as the body is at rest, the mitochondria in all the cells of the body, other than the brain, can produce energy entirely from fat. But they still rely heavily on glucose metabolism during times of exertion. Because of this, the mitochondrial energy deficit throughout the rest of the body will not be noticed until the body is exercised, in which case even minor exertion may seem too difficult.

A hallmark of early adrenal insufficiency is normal energy at rest with a substantial decrease in energy production during exercise. The hallmark for more severe states is fatigue both at rest and exertion.

❑ **Adrenal Insufficiency From Diet**

The adrenal glands - and your energy - also suffer from a diet too high in carbohydrate and too low in fat and protein.

In this respect, a strict vegetarian diet can inflict major harm on the adrenals. I have never seen total vegetarians (known as "vegans") who are healthy. And I've never seen one who is an athlete. It is just not compatible with optimum energy and performance.

Processed carbohydrates are particularly harmful to your ability to generate energy. By this I mean food items made with flour or white sugar, as well as refined rice, fruit juice, beer, and wine.

Carbohydrates such as these rapidly elevate your blood sugar, especially when consumed without adequate protein and fat.

From what I have already said about low blood sugar, you might think that elevated blood sugar is a good thing, but you'd be wrong. A high and/or rapidly rising blood sugar level causes the pancreas to secrete insulin, a hormone that acts to lower the blood sugar back down to normal.

However, if the adrenal glands are exhausted due to chronic stress, *and this condition is present in every ill person*, insulin causes the blood sugar to drop too far. Persistent intake of processed carbohydrates causes a sustained insulin production, which in turn exhausts the adrenal glands. Thus, we can say that high blood sugar often results in low blood sugar...and all the symptoms associated with it.

❑ The Wrong Fatty Acids

Special "gateway" sites on the surface of the cells called membrane receptors must be functional in order for cells to take in oxygen, fat, glucose, hormones, and nutrients critical to cellular activities, including energy production.

Receptors are extremely complicated structures and not much is

known about them. One thing we do know is that they are very much affected by the fatty acids that circulate in the blood. Fatty acids are the breakdown components of dietary fats.

Up until fifty or sixty years ago, Nature provided us with only one general category of fatty acids - called CIS fatty acids. These natural fatty acids are quite susceptible to oxidation and rancidity when separated out from their plant or animal origins.

When commercially processed foods began to proliferate, manufacturers needed to find a method to protect the fats they intended to use in their products. The method was to chemically treat the natural fatty acids with hydrogen in such a way that they were changed into stable fats with long shelf life and protection from rancidity. These man-made substitutes are called TRANS fatty acids.

Keep in mind that up until this point TRANS fatty acids never existed! They are completely foreign to the human body.

You can identify these substances by looking at ingredient labels where they are referred to as "hydrogenated" or "partially hydrogenated" oils of various kinds. *They are all harmful to our cells and undermine the integrity of membrane receptors*.

Since nothing gets into our cells except through these receptor sites, a diet high in trans fatty acids will markedly affect how cells function, and this will most notably be seen in how efficiently our mitochondria can utilize oxygen.

❑ Insufficient Fat Utilization

As I've already mentioned, all cells with the major exception of the brain cells, prefer burning fat for energy rather than carbohydrates (glucose). This is an important point because most people have been led to believe that optimum energy production comes from carbohydrates. Not so. **Optimum energy production is much more dependent on fat utilization.** The body evolved this way because fat is more efficiently stored, and produces less acid waste products than carbohydrates.

We have been led to believe that dietary fat makes body fat. But this is only half the truth. In fact, both dietary carbohydrates as well as dietary fat make body fat.

It works like this: When we eat, only a fraction of the food is used immediately for energy. Most becomes stored as fat.

That's right. **If you eat carbohydrates, they get stored as fat, and if you eat fat it gets stored as fat**. Either way, your body will store the "energy content" of your foods as fat.

Remember, we humans evolved in situations where the next meal was always in question. Thousands of years ago we may easily have gone several days or longer without eating. That's why the body evolved a system of storing dietary calories as fat. When the food was available, we ate as much as we could, and then hung on until the next meal, using the stored fat for energy in the interim.

The body can very easily store fat, but certain imbalances may make it hard to convert the stored fat to energy. The ability to break down stored fat and get it to the mitochondria for energy production is referred to as *fat utilization*.

Poor fat utilization leads to poor mitochondrial oxygen utilization and hence a lowered E.Q. If the body can't readily make use of its fat stores, it will do the next best thing and raid its reserves of carbohydrates. The problem here is that the body can only store a very small amount of carbohydrates. Within a matter of hours, the carbohydrate reserves become exhausted. This results in a falling blood sugar level.

And when the blood sugar level threatens to bottom out, the adrenal glands try to restore normalcy. If this scenario is repeated too often, it will ultimately stress the adrenal glands and cause adrenal insufficiency as I have described above.

The bottom line here is that excessive dietary carbohydrate - *and not fat* - leads to poor oxygen utilization, decreased mitochondrial function, and weight gain.

❑ Carnitine Deficiency

The early humans ate a diet high in meat. This meant an abundant intake of a vital amino acid called carnitine. Amino acids are the components of protein.

Researchers estimate that early man took in around 5,000 to 10,000 milligrams of carnitine per day. Currently, the average intake among Westerners is something like 100 milligrams.

Why? Carnitine is found only in animal fat and protein, and our modern dietary habits have shifted heavily towards carbohydrate with a smaller intake of animal protein and fat.

In the body, carnitine is converted into an enzyme called carnitine transferase, which is responsible for transporting the fat stores into the mitochondria for energy production. A deficiency of this enzyme, common nowadays because of carbohydrate-heavy diets, compromises your fat burning capability.

This will be reflected in decreased mitochondrial function and poor oxygen utilization. Signs of carnitine deficiency include fatigue and weight gain, combined with elevated triglycerides in the blood.

❑ Vitamin and Mineral Deficiencies

Once fat and/or glucose are introduced into the mitochondria, they enter into an assembly line process that eventually produces energy. First, in what is called the Krebs Cycle (also known as the Citric Acid Cycle), hydrogen atoms are removed from the fat and glucose molecules. This step requires optimum amounts of key amino acids, vitamins, and minerals, nutrients typically depleted when the body is stressed or the diet is poor. The most important nutrients are the B vitamins, especially niacin, B6, and riboflavin, along with the minerals magnesium and chromium.

❑ Coenzyme Q10 Deficiency

Coenzyme Q10, called CoQ10 for short, is a vitamin-like substance that is absolutely necessary for cellular energy production. After the Krebs cycle removes the hydrogen atoms from fat and glucose, they are combined with oxygen. This step, called cellular respiration, is where oxygen is turned into energy. The first and most critical enzyme in this process is CoQ10. As we age, we become deficient in CoQ10. Additionally, poor diet can also contribute to a deficiency. A deficiency will greatly limit your E.Q.

Chapter 3
Bio-Energy Testing™

Before you can effectively start increasing your E.Q., optimizing your energy production, and extending the length and quality of your life, the first step is to learn exactly how good (or bad) your present energy level is, and determine where problems lie.

Additionally, once you get started on your re-energizing program, you will want to objectively test the effectiveness of the program.

Why wait until some time off in the future to find out you were missing a few crucial steps and didn't realize your energetic potential?

The most reliable way by far to determine your needs and how well the program is working for you is through a complete metabolic and physiological assessment I call Bio-Energy Testing™.

Until recently there has not been a method to assess E.Q. accurately without an arterial puncture. This latter method, however, is painful, carries some degree of risk, and does not provide nearly as much useful information regarding energy production as does Bio-Energy Testing™.

Thanks to this unique test it is now possible to measure E.Q. easily, accurately, safely, and non-invasively, and for the first time accurately determine your metabolic rate and biological age. **This technology has enabled me to discover and verify the importance and efficacy of all the secrets of anti-aging presented in this book**.

Each secret has been found to improve E.Q. and biological age. That literally means slowing down and even reversing the aging process. I know this not because I read about it somewhere, or because it sounds like a really good theory. I know the secrets work because I have documented each of their effects with Bio-Energy Testing™.

You may be wondering: "What does he mean by biological age?"

Well, we know that chronological age simply refers to how many years you have been alive. Your biological age, on the other hand, refers to how old you are from a functional standpoint.

In the world of anti-aging medicine, chronological age is unimportant. It's your biological age that's important. That's what indicates how healthy you are, how well you feel and function, and how long you will likely live.

Many anti-aging specialists use various combinations of measurements to determine biological age. Such measurements include blood pressure, cholesterol levels, and lung function studies, just to name a few.

The problem is that all these methods have some flaws that limit their usefulness.

My research has shown me that biological age can most accurately be determined from E.Q. For example, a 75-year-old woman who has the E.Q. of a 45-year- old woman has a biological age of 45. And, in every case I have seen over the years, she will function every bit as well as a 45-year-old woman. Similarly, a 45-year-old woman with an E.Q. of a 75-year-old, has a biological age of 75, and consistently experiences symptoms characteristic of that older age group.

"But Doc, Is This Really Working?"

Before discovering the advantages of Bio-Energy Testing™, I, like other anti-aging physicians, had to just assume that the measures I was recommending to my patients were in fact really slowing down and reversing the aging process. Now, using the interpretations explained in this book, it is possible to actually demonstrate the effectiveness of these programs.

Bio-Energy Testing™ offers the most efficient and accurate health, aging, and fitness assessment available. It can quantitatively diagnose a decrease or increase in E.Q., as well as pinpoint whether an energy problem is located in the lungs, heart, arteries, capillaries, or mitochondria.

This information is essential to establishing an anti-aging program that maximizes your energy production, and also monitors its effectiveness.

Bio-Energy Testing™ is the ultimate tool for medical diagnostics, anti-aging medicine, weight management, and personal fitness training.

When you are evaluated with Bio-Energy Testing™ you will have the following critical metabolic measurements determined:

❏ Your M-Factor (your metabolism factor)

❏ Your C-Factor (your carbohydrate factor)

❏ Your FBR (exercise zone for maximum fat burning)

❏ Your Fat-Power Factor (how well you covert fat to power)

❑ Your ATR (exercise zone for optimum aerobic capacity)

❑ Your E.Q. (energy quotient)

❑ Your Biological Age (your "real" age)

❑ Your Fitness Factor (your overall fitness level)

I will show you in this book how these measurements are used to fine tune your disease prevention and anti-aging program, to improve your overall function, and to help you increase your energy levels.

The ABC's of Bio-Energy Testing™

❑ What the test involves

Bio-Energy Testing™ involves the use of a mouthpiece coupled with measuring devices that are able to measure how much oxygen the body uses and how much carbon dioxide the body is producing at any given time. A series of measurements is taken at rest and during exercise. I will describe these various measurements in a moment along with other important information that can help you live longer and healthier.

❑ What Bio-Energy Testing™ tells you

Your E.Q.

Your Biological age

Fitness level

Optimum dietary fat/carbohydrate ratio

Basal metabolic rate

Optimal exertion level for fat loss

Optimum exertion level for cardiovascular fitness

Metabolic health status

True anaerobic threshold

Hormonal imbalances

Causes of chronic fatigue states

❑ Who benefits from the test?

Anyone interested in slowing down the aging process

Anyone who wants to feel and function like a much younger person

Chronically-fatigued individuals

Anyone needing help with weight control

Anyone interested in preventing the diseases of aging

Anyone with heart disease, diabetes, arthritis, or high cholesterol

People who want to know if their anti-aging program is working

Anyone involved in cardiovascular exercise

Anyone desiring to maximize workout efficiency

❑ Where to get the test

To obtain the name of a facility in your area offering Bio-Energy Testing™, please go to www.bursting-with-energy.com, or call 1-866-376-0610.

❑ How much does it cost?

The cost for Bio-Energy Testing™ will vary depending on where you have it performed, but typically runs in the area of $200 - $250.

Preliminaries To Bio-Energy Testing™

Here are some tips and insights you should know prior to testing.

Elderly persons and individuals with heart disease should be cleared by their physician before undertaking the exercise portion of the test.

Healthy persons, particularly those already exercising, can take the test without reservation.

The resting part of the test is performed in the morning before 10:30 AM. You should not eat or drink anything other than water. Be extremely lazy before the test. Both physical and mental exertion should be kept to a minimum, and definitely, no exercise.

Record your resting heart rate for several days prior to the test. This is accomplished by wearing a heart rate monitor to bed. Heart rate monitors can be purchased at bicycle shops and sporting good stores, and usually cost around $100. They come equipped with a strap outfitted with an electrode that you adhere to your chest over the heart. You read your heart rate on a monitor that looks like a watch.

Just before bedtime, attach the electrode. Place the monitor on a bedside stand so that you can read it in the morning without having to sit up or reach over. In other words, with little effort.

When you wake up, check your heart rate on the monitor with as little motion as possible. If you had a restless night, or if you were up to the bathroom within three hours of waking, do not use the measurement.

In this manner, record your resting heart rate for several mornings and bring the log to your testing facility. The readings should be very similar. For most people, the reading will be between 55 and 70 beats per minute.

People in better condition will have lower readings. Some athletes may have a resting heart rate of less than 40.

The First Test: Basal Testing

After you arrive at the testing center, the technician will record your height and weight. Next, a heart rate monitor will be strapped to your chest and you will be placed in a comfortable reclining chair. You should be relaxed, mentally and physically. Do not be concerned about the outcome of the test.

Failure to adequately relax can influence the basal measurements.

Within a few minutes of settling down in the chair, the technician places a mouthpiece in your mouth. You will be instructed to ignore the device and just continue to take it easy. There is no discomfort, so relaxing shouldn't be a problem.

As you just lay back and relax, the analyzer determines your resting oxygen intake and carbon dioxide output.

Exercise Testing

After this initial resting measurement the fun really begins.

You are placed on an ergometer, a fancy name for an exercise bicycle that uses a computer to measure how hard you are working. The seat of the cycle is adjusted so that your leg is straight when the heel of your foot is on the pedal in the most extended position.

The technician again gives you the measuring mouthpiece to place in your mouth. Now you will begin to cycle.

It is important to use a correct technique. This is accomplished simply enough by doing what is referred to as "pedaling in circles." You make as much an effort to lift on the up stroke as when you push down on the down stroke. This technique allows you to generate more power from your legs for the test.

For the first several minutes, very little effort is required. Then the workload on the ergometer will gradually increase so that you will have to work harder to turn the pedals. As the level of exertion increases your heart rate will also increase.

The test continues until the technician notifies you that you have entered into anaerobic energy production. At this point the test is concluded.

How The Bio-Energy Testing™ Analyzer "Knows"

Imagine a salesperson trying to convince a prospective buyer to buy a thermos.

"If you put something cold into it," he says, "it will stay cold. If you put in something hot, it will stay hot."

The man buys the thermos and then comes back a few weeks later.

"There's no problem at all with the thermos," he says happily. "It works great. It keeps hot things hot and cold things cold, but what I don't understand is how does it know?"

In order for you to understand how the Bio-Energy Testing™ analyzer "knows," we'll take a short tour through some of the measurements used in Bio-Energy Testing™, and how they relate to the process of energy production in the body. This information can get incredibly complex, but I've attempted to keep it as simple as possible.

Your Respiratory Quotient (RQ)

Oxygen is an extremely high-energy molecule. Animals, including humans, convert oxygen, which is Nature's highest energy molecule, to water, which is Nature's lowest energy molecule. In this process, energy is released. **It is this energy that powers every aspect of your life**!

This process also generates carbon dioxide as a waste product in direct proportion to the amount of energy released.

Since all the oxygen enters the body through the lungs, and all the carbon dioxide is eliminated from the lungs, the energy conversion process can be gauged by measuring how much oxygen and carbon dioxide are coming in and going out with each breath you take. That's precisely what the Bio-Energy Testing™ analyzer does.

The mouthpiece in the analyzer contains sophisticated transducers capable of accurately measuring both oxygen and carbon dioxide as you breathe in and out. The ratio of oxygen going in to carbon dioxide coming out reflects how efficiently your body produces energy.

Let's say that the Bio-Energy Testing™ analyzer determines you are releasing only a small amount of carbon dioxide in relation to the amount of oxygen you are breathing in. This tells us you are converting only a small amount of oxygen to energy.

Or let's say that your body eliminates a high level of carbon dioxide relative to the amount of oxygen being consumed. This tells us there is an increased conversion of oxygen to energy.

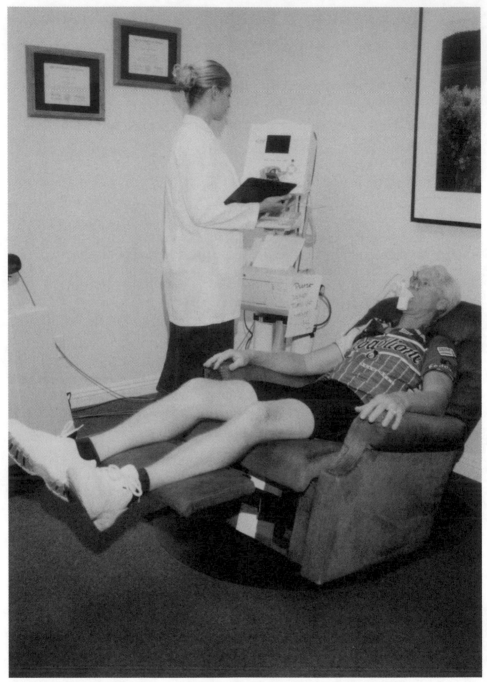

Bio-Energy Testing: *In a recent test, Dr. Shallenberger's measurements indicated low metabolism and a need to increase his thyroid supplementation.*

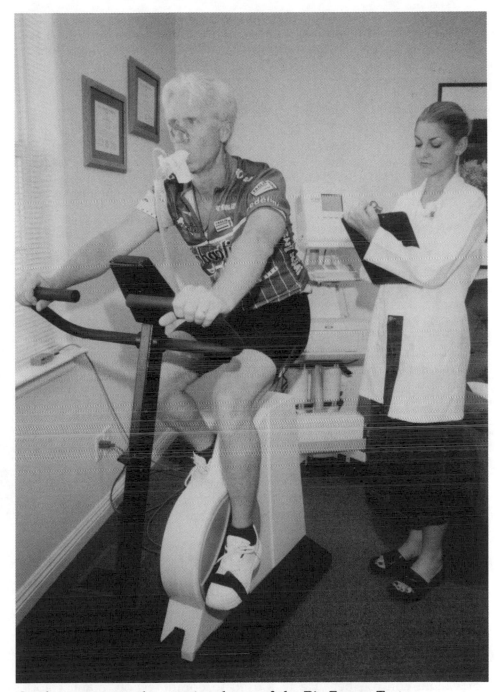

On the ergometer, the exertional part of the Bio-Energy Test:
Dr. Shallenberger's "energy quotient" results were the equivalent of a forty-year old. Not bad for a baby boomer!

Thus, the ratio of carbon dioxide produced to oxygen consumed is a direct indicator of how much energy your body is producing. This ratio is called the respiratory quotient or RQ.

The RQ Equation

Oxygen + fat or carbohydrate ⇨ carbon dioxide + water + ENERGY

RQ = Amount carbon dioxide/Amount oxygen

Bio-Energy Testing™ At A Glance

Bio-Energy Testing™ determines your RQ at rest and at various stages of work performed. Using this information, the computer then calculates your M-Factor (reflecting your metabolism), your C-Factor (whether you are producing energy from carbohydrate or fat), your FBR (fat burning heart rate), your Fat-Power Factor (how efficiently your fat stores work for you), your ATR (anaerobic threshold heart rate), your Fitness Factor (your level of fitness), your E.Q. (energy quotient), and your biological ("real") age.

You need to be familiar with these measurements in order to properly understand and appreciate how valuable Bio-Energy Testing™ can be to your health and longevity.

Each of these values are important parameters to determine how healthy you are, the quality of your diet, the efficiency of your exercise program, how well your anti-aging program is working for you, and, ultimately, how well you produce energy.

These measurements are discussed below.

Your M-Factor (Metabolic Factor)

By measuring your oxygen consumption at rest the Bio-Energy Testing™ analyzer determines your basal metabolic rate (BMR). This is a measurement of your level of energy production at rest, and is a reflection of your overall metabolism. Persons with a high BMR have high metabolic rates, and those with a low BMR have low metabolic rates.

Besides being an overall health factor, your BMR is especially valuable for weight control, because it is used to compute how many calories your body will burn in a day.

There are many formulas designed to estimate BMR, but for most people, especially those for whom it is the most important, these estimates are almost always inaccurate. Bio-Energy Testing™ allows us to precisely measure your exact BMR. More importantly, once your BMR is measured we can determine your M-Factor.

For persons younger than forty, the M-Factor is equal to the ratio of their measured BMR, as determined by Bio-Energy Testing™ compared to the average BMR of healthy persons the same age, weight, and gender.

For those over forty, the M-Factor equals the ratio of the measured BMR compared to the average BMR of healthy forty year olds the same weight and gender.

The Optimum M-Factor is 100 percent.

M-Factor declines linearly with aging. It is therefore an excellent yardstick of your rate of aging. It is not only an excellent way to determine how well your anti-aging program is working, but also supplies critical information needed to establish the correct therapeutic program for optimum energy production and weight control.

The M-Factor also declines with disease, and varies considerably from person to person based upon genetics, hormone levels (particularly thyroid and adrenal hormones), muscle mass, fitness, and diet. Nutrient deficiencies, especially B-vitamins, magnesium, fatty acids, and coenzyme Q10, can also play a significant role in determining the M-Factor.

Your M-Factor can signal significant decreases in thyroid function (hypothyroidism) that might otherwise go undiagnosed. A low M-Factor is the most sensitive indicator of low thyroid states even when thyroid blood tests show normal values. The thyroid discussion in my Secret No. 8 - natural hormone replacement - goes into more detail on this important matter.

Your C-Factor

Your C-Factor determines whether your energy is coming from the metabolism of fat or carbohydrate. This is an important detail because energy produced from fat creates less carbon dioxide than energy produced from carbohydrate. The reason for this relates to the different amount of oxygen and carbon dioxide contained in the molecular makeup of fat and carbohydrate.

For example, each glucose molecule (what all carbohydrates ultimately break down to) produces six molecules of carbon dioxide from six molecules of oxygen. If you remember that RQ = carbon dioxide/oxygen, you will note that this means an RQ equal to one. **Thus, when the**

Bio-Energy Testing™ analyzer measures your RQ to be equal to 1, that means your body is producing its energy purely from carbohydrate. No fat is being metabolized at all.

Fat molecules are different however, and each fat molecule produces sixteen molecules of carbon dioxide from twenty-three molecules of oxygen for an RQ of 16/23 or .70.

So when the Bio-Energy Testing™ analyzer determines your RQ as .70, that indicates you are burning purely fat and no carbohydrate.

Fat's lower RQ ratio translates to *30 percent less carbon dioxide production* produced by fat metabolism than by carbohydrate.

Since carbon dioxide is an *acid*, we say that fat metabolism results in a cleaner, healthier form of energy production than carbohydrate metabolism because it generates less carbon dioxide and hence less acid. Excessive tissue acid production is considered a hallmark of all chronic disease, and anything that decreases it is considered highly beneficial. Efficient fat metabolism decreases acid production and is why it is so essential to your health. Both your C-Factor and your Fat-Power Factor (I'll discuss this later) measure how efficiently you metabolize fat.

Optimum C-Factor

The optimal RQ in a resting state is between .72 and .78. That's what is typically measured in healthy young people. This means that at rest they are producing virtually all of their energy from fat. As you learned a moment ago, if they produced all their energy from fat, the RQ would be .70.

The reason they don't produce 100 percent of their energy from fat relates to the brain. Unlike every other organ in the body the brain can only utilize carbohydrate for energy, and since the brain is still quite active even in a resting state, the carbohydrate metabolism going on in the brain raises the RQ slightly.

Most of the time when I measure a resting RQ for a new patient the result is much higher than the optimal range of .72-.78. This finding is very significant. **Values higher than .78 are caused by excessive dietary carbohydrate, because dietary carbohydrate decreases the body's ability to burn fa**t. This impact on fat metabolism is the ultimate cause of obesity and many other diseases and health problems. I'll talk more about this later on when I explain my secrets for weight management and disease prevention.

Your C-Factor is your measured resting RQ multiplied by 100. It tells you whether or not your diet contains the optimum ratio of fat, carbohydrate, and protein. An optimum C-Factor is between 72-78.

The bottom line on your C-Factor is this: if it is greater than 78, you need to decrease your intake of carbohydrate and optimize your exercise program to burn fat more efficiently. How much should carbs be cut back? This varies greatly from person to person. In some cases almost all dietary carbs must be eliminated. Bio EnergyTesting™ gives us the individual answer. The reduction must be sufficient enough to bring the C-Factor back to 78 or lower.

A C-Factor greater than 90 is not uncommon, and indicates a much more serious impediment to fat metabolism than simply too much dietary carbohydrate. More than 90 means the presence of a serious energy deficit disorder that often requires therapeutic detoxification and/or hormonal replacement in order to normalize energy production. Not optimizing the C-Factor leaves an individual especially vulnerable to premature aging and degenerative diseases, and makes it difficult, if not impossible, to lose weight.

Your FBR (Fat Burning Heart Rate)

Are you keeping up so far?

Just remember that your M-Factor directly correlates with aging, and can signal significant decreases in metabolism and thyroid function (hypothyroidism) that might otherwise go undiagnosed. Your M-Factor should ideally equal 100 percent.

And don't forget that in a resting state your body should be primarily using fat as its energy fuel. This is reflected in an optimal C-Factor below 78. If you eat too much carbohydrate, you are interfering with optimal fat-to-energy conversion, as well as causing increased tissue acid accumulation. In that case you will have a C-Factor above 78.

From here let's proceed from the resting state into activity. And into exercise. As you begin to start exercising, some interesting metabolic changes begin to occur

Although fat is a cleaner, less toxic form of energy fuel, it is carbohydrate that is actually a more efficient producer of energy. Additionally, its chemical structure renders it more readily available when the demand for energy rises. Thus, as the work load on the ergometer gradually increases and your energy demands increase, your body will begin to progressively burn more carbohydrate. And as your body burns more carbohydrate your RQ will correspondingly rise. Eventually, as the testing continues, your RQ will reach .85. This is the point where the body is burning the maximum amount of fat possible for energy production.

I refer to the *heart rate* at this point as the **fat burning heart rate, or FBR**. When you are exercising at your FBR, your body is burning fat as fast as it can. As your exercise intensity drives your heart rate beyond your FBR, the proportion of energy produced from fat metabolism progressively declines, and your energy needs begin to rely on burning ever-increasing amounts of carbohydrate. Another way of putting it is to say that to the degree that you are exercising either below or above your FBR, you are burning less than maximal amounts of fat. This is why knowing your actual FBR, not one "guesstimated" from a formula, is so vitally important for those needing to get better control of their weight.

Your Fat-Power Factor

One of the most fantastic aspects of Bio-Energy Testing™ is that it is able to accurately measure how much work is being performed during the exercise portion of the test. In this context the word "work" refers to a scientific measurement of how much power is being generated.

A good example of the concept of work can be found in the way we use the word horsepower to describe the power output of an engine. Obviously, the higher the engine's horsepower, the stronger that engine is, and the more work it can do.

Your Fat-Power Factor refers to the maximum amount of work that your body can generate purely from fat. If you are forty-years old or younger, the Fat Power Factor compares you to people your same age. If you are older than forty, the Fat Power Factor compares you to a forty-year old your same weight and gender.

The higher your Fat-Power Factor, the more power you are able to produce from fat. A Fat-Power Factor greater than or equal to 100 is optimal because it indicates that your body is utilizing fat as an energy source with the maximum efficiency possible.

Are You Burning Fat Efficiently?

Dietary fat has received an enormous amount of negative press over the years. Yet fat is absolutely central to energy production.

My use of Bio-Energy Testing™ has taught me an amazing fact: a decline in fat metabolism is more responsible for the effects of aging than any other single factor. This is because fat is the body's ideal energy raw material. Nature designed it that way.

To reiterate what's been said before, every time we eat, the energy from the meal is stored as fat. That is, *both* carbohydrates and fats become *stored as fat*.

Remember that our bodies have evolved over many thousands of years, and our ancestors were never quite sure of their next meal. Three squares a day has become a reality for humans only in our modern age. We still have caveman bodies living in a supermarket world, but the evolutionary process of storing meals as fat has not changed. The stored fat is still intended to fuel energy production during the time between meals.

Thus, if your body cannot burn fat efficiently, you not only gain weight, you have low energy production as well. And the resultant low energy only serves to speed the aging process at an ever-increasing rate. **Aging, gaining weight, and low energy all go hand in hand.** They're just different sides of the same problem - an inability to burn or metabolize fat. Proof of this is the fact that an increase in body fat composition is universally regarded as one of reliable indicator of the aging process.

Despite what you hear from many "experts" in the diet industry, it is excessive carbohydrate consumption - and not fat - that is the major dietary cause of weight gain. It also is the leading cause of diabetes and high cholesterol.

In my practice, less than one in twenty patients puts on weight by eating too much fat.

It seems like a reasonable enough assumption that eating fat causes fat gain, but the science doesn't support such an assumption for the majority of people.

Certainly, one of the most useful aspects of Bio-Energy Testing™ is that it can determine both your C-Factor and your Fat-Power Factor. These measurements can specifically tell you how well you metabolize fat, how much power your body can generate from fat, and hence how fast you are aging.

People unable to lose weight often have a Fat-Power Factor significantly less than 100, along with a C-Factor greater than 85. Functionally speaking, that means their entire daily energy needs are being met by carbohydrate metabolism. No wonder they can't lose weight. **They can't burn fat!**

For these people, any form of exercise is very limited for fat burning purposes, because fat burning metabolism is already maxed out at rest!

Such people tell me that no matter how hard they exercise they can't lose weight. Only when the causes of their metabolic imbalances are corrected can they burn fat effectively during exertion, and thus lose undesirable weight.

Optimum fat metabolism as indicated by an optimum C-Factor and Fat-Power Factor accomplishes a great number of other very desirable effects in addition to weight control, including:

❑ Decreasing your rate of aging.

❑ Reducing the level of metabolic acids that contribute to chronic disease.

❑ Increasing your endurance.

❑ Increasing your energy levels.

❑ Maintaining your blood sugar levels.

❑ Lowering your blood fats - cholesterol and triglycerides

Your ATR (Anaerobic Threshold Heart Rate)

We still have you on the ergometer, the cycling machine that is giving the Bio-Energy Testing™ your "vital statistics."

As the testing continues, and the ergometer gradually increases your exertion level, your heart rate increases beyond your FBR. Because more and more carbohydrate is being burned to meet your energy requirements, your RQ also increases.

Eventually you reach an RQ equal to 1.0.

An RQ of 1.0, you'll remember, signifies that the total energy needs are being met entirely by carbohydrate. No fat is burned at all when an RQ of 1.0 is reached. Only carbohydrate.

This point is called the **anaerobic threshold, or AT, and it indicates the point of maximum energy production from oxygen.**

All energy produced beyond your AT is produced without oxygen, i.e., anaerobic metabolism. Anaerobic metabolism as we have seen, is undesirable.

As I mentioned before, it is easy to feel the effects of anaerobic metabolism first hand. Simply hold your breath. You will almost immediately go into a state of 100 percent anaerobic metabolism. It will take you less than a minute of holding your breath to figure out a few things about anaerobic metabolism:

❑ It can only meet your energy demands for a very limited amount of time. As I mentioned earlier, this is because the production of energy in the body from anaerobic metabolism is only a fraction of that produced when oxygen is used.

❑ The brain panics and eventually becomes non-functional. This is because it is the most sensitive organ to energy deficiency states.

❑ It hurts! This because anaerobic metabolism produces a huge amount of lactic acid, and excessive lactic acid causes pain in the muscles.

❏ You become breathless. This is because anaerobic metabolism causes a buildup of carbon dioxide. This is what drives your breathing rate.

Not only does anaerobic metabolism feel discomforting, but it is also as bad for you as it feels. It causes increasing free radical damage in the body, puts the adrenal glands into a hyper state, and creates a high tide of acid in the tissues.

Now imagine a person who has a low AT. This means that they will go into anaerobic metabolism, and experience all the above symptoms, even at very low levels of exertion.

Over the years I have been astounded to see many patients with AT's so low that they go into anaerobic metabolism simply by walking across the room! These persons are commonly labeled with chronic fatigue syndrome or fibromyalgia. They complain of profound fatigue, mental confusion, anxiety and panic states, muscle aches and pains, and breathlessness and lack of endurance. Unless the causes of decreased AT are successfully addressed, their lives are quite limited.

I refer to your heart rate when you reach AT as your **ATR, or anaerobic threshold heart rate.** Don't confuse that with an **ATM.**

Your E.Q.

As you have learned, the body can make energy in two ways, aerobically and anaerobically. The maximum total possible energy production therefore is the sum of these two. This sum is lower in smaller persons and in older persons, and because of the influence of estrogen, it is also lower in women than in men.

Your E.Q. is the amount of energy your body can produce aerobically (i.e., when you reach your AT), compared to an estimated maximum total energy production. The estimated maximum total energy production that is used for this comparison is determined by testing the total energy production of hundreds of healthy men and women of various ages and weights, and finding the average.

If you are forty-years old or younger, your E.Q. compares you to people your same gender, age, and weight. If you are older than forty, the E.Q. compares you to a forty-year old with your same gender, age, and weight.

Your E.Q is a global measurement that reflects the sum total of all the factors involved in energy production including hemoglobin, lung function, heart strength, circulation, 2,3 DPG, fat metabolism, carbohydrate metabolism, and mitochondrial efficiency. Obviously, if any of these factors is less than optimal, it will result in a decreased E.Q. So the E.Q is a cross check on *all* the physiological functions required to make energy.

An E.Q. equal to or greater than 100 is the goal. It would mean you are readily generating a substantial amount of energy with the greatest possible efficiency.

Moreover, it means that no matter how old you are, your body is producing energy as effectively as a 40-year-old. I'll explain the importance of this last statement in the next few paragraphs when I discuss the concept of biological age.

E.Q. levels falling below 100 indicate the degree that aging and lifestyle factors are robbing you of perfect health. Low E.Q.'s are associated with decreased energy and stamina, and a decreased ability to perform and function optimally across the board.

The Ferrari And The Clunker

To illustrate my point, let's turn to the automotive world for a moment, and put you behind the wheel of a brand new Ferrari.

The tank is filled with the highest-octane gasoline available to accommodate the high performance engine. The fuel pump and the carburetor are delivering the gas to the cylinders. The spark plugs are new. The battery has plenty of juice.

This is analogous to you having good lungs, a good heart, and good circulation.

Everything is set for a great ride.

But what if the engine is out of tune? That new Ferrari will run no better than an old clunker. In fact, a well-tuned old clunker may outperform a poorly tuned new Ferrari.

When your body is tuned, your E.Q. will be 100 or higher. Nothing is more tied to good mental and physical functioning and disease prevention than optimum energy production through an optimum E.Q.

Your Biological Age: How Old Are You Really?

Alas, but energy production steadily decreases with age. The decline results in diminished function in every single cell, tissue, and organ in the body, and is the modus operandi behind the symptoms of aging.

Since the brain and the heart are the largest consumers of energy in the body, it is these organs that are the most affected. But no part of your body is spared. That's the bad news.

The good news is that you may be a clunker chronologically, but you have the potential to perform like a new Ferrari.

A successful anti-aging program can prevent and often reverse a declining E.Q. **Alternatively, if your program doesn't optimize your E.Q., or at the very least halt the decline, it is not working!**

Determining your E.Q. is one more reason why Bio-Energy Testing™ technology is so vital. It tells you your biological age, that is, the age at which your body is functioning.

You are as functionally old as your E.Q. Increase your E.Q. and you decrease your biological age. You become more functionally youthful.

The Bio-Energy Testing™ analyzer can determine your biological age by seeing how your E.Q. result matches up with healthy individuals of different ages. For example, if your E.Q. is equal to 100, your biological age is forty or less no matter how old you are chronologically. Similarly, if it is equal to fifty, your biological age is eighty years old!

So now, no matter how many candles they stick in your birthday cake, by determining your biological age, you can know how old you *really* are!

Your Fitness Factor

Remember that your Fat Power Factor tells you how well your body is converting fat to work. On the other hand, your Fitness Factor tells you how well your body is converting both fat *and* carbohydrate to work. It therefore refers to the maximum total amount of work that your body is able to perform aerobically.

The Fitness Factor is a function of E.Q. but differs because it also takes into consideration your *overall strength*. E.Q. measures how well you make energy. Fitness factor measures how well your muscles convert that energy into power.

If you are forty-years old or younger, the Fitness Factor compares you to people your same age. If you are older than forty, the Fitness Factor compares you to a forty-year old with your same weight and gender.

The higher your Fitness Factor, the more total power your body is able to produce. A Fitness Factor greater than or equal to 100 is optimal because it indicates that your body is producing power with the maximum efficiency possible.

Now that you are familiar with the importance of these vital Bio-Energy Testing™ measurements, let's move on and introduce you to the practical steps you can take to improve each and every reading.

Chapter 4
Energy and Detoxification

Why do some people age so much more rapidly than others? You've no doubt wondered about that as you've watched friends and relatives over the years.

The basic reason, as we've seen, is that those who age faster are unable to generate adequate levels of energy. This is reflected in sub-optimal Bio-Energy Testing™ measurements.

Aside from genetics, one of the greatest factors influencing the decrease in energy production is toxicity. By toxicity, I mean the progressive accumulation of harmful substances, referred to as toxins, in the cells and tissues of the body.

Toxins can certainly come from the environment in the form of heavy metals, food additives, pharmaceuticals, cigarettes, and chemicals. Surprisingly, however, the overwhelming source of toxicity is our very own bodies.

Each and every cell in our body takes in oxygen and nutrients, and from these substances produces energy *and* waste products. The wastes materialize in the form of organic acids. They are very toxic, and must be moved out of the system in order for us to maintain health.

Other sources of toxicity in the body include the mouth, the sinuses, and the bowels. I'll discuss these in a moment.

Regardless of the source, the important thing to remember is that **toxins decrease cellular energy production.** Since the very tissues and organs that are responsible for treatment and removal of bodily toxins require substantial energy production themselves, a vicious cycle is created resulting in a persistent decline in energy production as we become older and more toxic.

All the "secrets" I'll be sharing with you in part two relate in some way to detoxification and improving your energy level. Before I begin giving you the practical how-to information, let me take a moment to discuss toxicity and toxin removal in the body.

Your Internal Sewer

It's not a very pleasant scene down in the lower intestine after the remnants of food have passed through the digestive and absorption processes. Basically, you're looking at an internal sewer, teeming with bacterial and fungal life, putrefied matter, incompletely digested foods, pesticides, dyes, preservatives, and probably a fair share of parasites.

Your body deals with this mess in a number of ways. First and foremost, more than 90 percent of your immune system activity occurs in the intestinal tract where immune cells constantly battle foreign "invaders" and toxins. This activity requires a huge amount of energy to keep up the job. But as good as the immune system is, it can't prevent all the bowel toxins from finding their way into the bloodstream.

Fortunately there is a back up system. Before the blood that drains the intestines enters into the general circulation, it passes through the liver where the toxins are filtered out. Fortunately, I say, because if this were not the case, you would die within a matter of hours. That's how important the detoxifying power of the liver is to your health!

As long as the liver is able to function optimally, it can effectively protect the rest of the body from the negative effects of these toxins. The liver, too, requires an enormous amount of energy production to accomplish its critical janitorial services. Illness and the aging process erode this energy production, and liver function suffers. As a result, more toxic materials, many of them carcinogenic, are able to get through and into the general circulation.

Oral Toxins

Dr. Gary Verigin is a friend and internationally respected biological dentist. A biological dentist is one who appreciates and understands how dramatically our dental health affects overall health. Dr. Verigin long ago told me, "that the routine use in dentistry of silver amalgam fillings is a major source of toxicity in the human body." My experience working with patients with various health disorders has abundantly confirmed this statement.

Since the late 1800s, dentists have been using "silver" amalgam fillings as the preferred treatment for cavities. Many years ago I was shocked to learn that 50 percent of these amalgams are comprised of the extremely toxic heavy metal mercury. One average size amalgam filling contains about 780 milligrams of mercury, enough to exceed the U.S. Environmental Protection Agency's mercury intake standard for one person for 100 years!

Of course dentists have always thought that once amalgam fillings were mixed and put in place, the mercury was somehow "locked" in. Several years ago however, researchers learned that this is not the case. Studies revealed that mercury vapor is continuously released in the mouth by the activity of chewing, brushing, and drinking hot liquids. Thus, patients with amalgams are constantly exposed to mercury every day.

Mercury is extremely toxic, more so than lead, cadmium, or arsenic. Other than fluoride, it is the most toxic of all naturally occurring substances. Organic mercury, called methyl mercury, and the inorganic form found in the vapor from amalgams are the most toxic forms. **There is no known non-toxic level for mercury vapor**.

The vapor very easily enters the body, where levels build up with time. *Mercury is a potent suppressor of mitochondrial activity.* It damages brain and nerve tissue, the thyroid, pituitary, and adrenal glands, the heart and lungs, as well as hormones and enzymes.

Mercury depletes the immune system. One study found significant suppression of helper cells, vital components of the immune system, in each and every patient tested who had silver amalgams. The cells returned to a more normal status when the amalgams were removed. These cells become rapidly suppressed when silver amalgams are placed in patients who previously have no such fillings, according to the research.

Scientific findings also indicate that mercury vapor contributes to allergies and auto-immune disorders such as multiple sclerosis, lupus, and rheumatoid arthritis.

Other studies have revealed that ingested mercury released from fillings causes harmful yeast organisms commonly found in the intestines to become resistant to the defense mechanisms of the immune system.

Mercury easily penetrates the placental membrane and damages the brain and nervous system of unborn babies. For that reason, the American Dental Association has recommended that silver amalgam fillings not be placed in the mouths of pregnant women. What is ignored is the effect of the mercury fillings already in place in these women!

The Occupational Safety and Health Administration and the Environmental Protection Agency have declared leftover scrap dental amalgam as a toxic hazard to dental personnel, to the dental office, and to the environment. These agencies require very rigid protocols for the handling and disposal of the exact same dental material that is placed in your mouth!

Chronic mercury poisoning can affect all of the body tissues and mimic many common diseases. Many people recover from diseases after the fillings are removed, and the residual mercury is chelated (chemically removed) out of the body. The most prevalent signs and symptoms of chronic exposure to mercury are:

PSYCHOLOGICAL: Irritability, anxiety, depression, fits of anger, loss of self-control and self-confidence, nervousness, shyness or timidity, memory loss.

NEUROLOGIC: Chronic or frequent headaches, dizziness, speech difficulties, coordination difficulties, and tremors.

CARDIOVASCULAR: Irregular heartbeat, feeble and irregular pulse, alterations in blood pressure, pain and pressure in the chest.

RESPIRATORY: Persistent cough, shallow and irregular respiration, emphysema.

OTHER: Joint pains, muscle weakness, fatigue, anemia, allergies, metallic taste in mouth, excessive salivation, bleeding gums, foul breath, loosening of teeth and bone loss, excessive perspiration, cold and clammy skin, sub-normal temperature, edema, abdominal cramps, colitis, diarrhea.

Chronic Sinus Infections - Just Watch TV

Inflammation stemming from allergies and chronic sinus infections is a very common source of toxicity. All you have to do is watch TV for a couple of hours and count the sinus medication advertisements to know that this is really a big problem.

Foods and inhalants are the most common sources of allergies. Interestingly enough, as we age our allergies tend to disappear. This is because allergies are an overreaction of the immune system. The immune system requires a huge amount of energy to operate, and as we grow older and energy production declines, immunity declines as well, resulting in a decreased incidence of allergies. Nevertheless, long before the allergies have gone away, chronic sinus infections have often taken root, and a depressed immune system only makes them harder to eliminate.

The persistent use of antibiotics and antihistamines without judiciously removing the allergic offenders that caused the sinus infection in the first place only results in chronic sinus infections that become resistant to therapy. The immunological reactive materials such as free radicals, peroxides, immunoglobulins, and immune complexes that our immune system uses to fight these chronic infections are highly toxic and must be cleared by the liver.

As you can imagine, the liver, as one of the body's most metabolically active organs, is unable to clear these toxic reactive materials without solid energy production. Furthermore, these toxins actually react with the mitochondria in the liver and elsewhere to decrease energy production even more.

A dangerous vicious cycle develops as we age. Age related decrease in energy production in liver cells leads to decreased liver function, which results in higher levels of these toxic immune reactive materials throughout the body. The escalating level of these materials causes a further decrease in energy production by their negative effect on mitochondria.

This scenario can easily go on for decades and leads to a rising level of toxicity. In many cases the only treatments needed to clear these chronic sinus conditions are those which improve both energy production and liver function.

Detoxification To The Rescue

The process of eliminating toxins is referred to as detoxification. Without adequate detoxification, toxins accumulate in the tissues, and over many years the body becomes a veritable toxic waste dump!

Imagine how much efficiency is lost by organs trying to carry out their functions under the burden of a half-century's buildup of pollution and poison. It's easy to understand why they deteriorate at an accelerated rate. By understanding how your body eliminates these toxins, you will be able to assist it, and prevent toxin accumulation, and the inevitable decrease in energy production that comes from it.

❑ The Lymph System

The first step in the detoxification process occurs when the cells excrete their waste products into the lymph fluid.

Imagine the cells of your body aligned like a brick wall, but instead of cement, they are separated by fluid. This fluid is called the lymph fluid. The lymph fluid meanders through a network of lymph ducts, and eventually dumps its cargo of wastes into the blood stream just above the heart.

In order to assist this flow into the blood stream, two factors are required. One is movement, meaning activity in which we move the muscles of the arms and particularly the legs. I don't mean exercise, but just the routine walking and arm movements that occur in every day life. People who especially need to be aware of this are ones with sedentary jobs in which they sit for long periods of time, like truck drivers, writers, or office workers. If you work a job like this, be sure to get up every thirty minutes or so and walk around madly waving your arms. I'm kidding of course, but you get the idea.

The second factor is lying down. No problem there, huh?

I'll bet that you didn't realize that lying down was so vital to your health. Here we finally have a health concept that most everyone can handle. The under twenty age-group needs about ten hours of horizontal time per twenty-four hour cycle. Over twenty needs at least eight hours.

Lying down allows the lymph fluid to gravity drain. So when you sleep, the body is busy cleaning up the mess that was made during the day. Detoxification and repair are actually the primary activities of the body during sleep.

❑ The Kidneys

After the lymph fluid is dumped into the blood stream, the circulation carries the toxins to the kidneys and the liver. Certain toxins are selectively removed in the kidneys and dispatched to the bladder, where they are eliminated through the urine.

In order to do their jobs, the kidneys require water - pure water, and plenty of it. Not coffee. Not soda. Not juice. Not milk. In fact, these fluids may actually impede kidney function. Just water.

And water, as you will read later on, is one of my "secrets" for better health and energy.

❑ The Liver And Intestines

The toxins that aren't eliminated by the kidneys are processed in the liver and channeled into the intestinal tract. Here, dietary fiber acts like a sponge and absorbs the toxins, escorting them out of the body through the feces.

This is why fiber is so important. Fiber, I should point out, is the roughage in vegetables and whole grains. Your body doesn't absorb fiber. Instead, this material acts as a broom, keeping the intestines clean and carrying out the waste products removed by the liver.

People who eat diets high in processed, refined carbohydrates such as bread and pasta are often missing adequate fiber. They run the risk, among other harmful effects, of having toxins reabsorbed back into the body, which means the liver has to work harder.

Fiber also enhances regular bowel movements and helps to prevent constipation. Chronic constipation is a major cause of toxin accumulation in the tissues.

Your Liver: The Most Important Organ In The Body

The body is a dynamic, interacting organism. It is affected by even the slightest alterations in the environment, as well as by thought, emotion, and diet. Of course these influences are continually changing, and in the process they easily throw the body out of balance.

Not to worry, however. The body has a miraculous ability to diagnose and correct these imbalances as they occur.

This ability is handled by the body's homeostatic regulation systems. And nothing is more important to a healthy body than the optimal functioning of these systems, which are controlled by interactions between the brain and the liver.

These two organs are not only designed to correct homeostatic disturbances, but in fact actually require the disturbances. That's right, in order for your body to be fully healthy, it needs to be constantly challenged.

Most people would think that the most important homeostatic organ in the body is the brain. And it's true that the brain has the most direct incoming and outgoing connection with all the cells and organs in the body. But it's not the most important simply because it is largely invulnerable. The brain sits in its ivory tower like a general, separated and protected from most toxins and infections by what is known as the blood brain barrier. This barrier allows only a very select group of molecules to come into actual contact with the brain.

Contrast this with the liver. **Unlike the brain, the liver operates precisely where all toxins are directed.** The liver must clear virtually every toxin in the body, from bacteria and viruses to pesticides and metabolic waste products.

Not only that, but it is also responsible for processing the nutrients you eat. Every molecule you ingest, whether it is a vitamin, mineral, fat, protein, or carbohydrate, must first be processed by the liver before being used by the cells of the body.

Additionally, the liver regulates the balance of all the protein, fat, and carbohydrate in the blood. In combination with the spleen and intestines, the liver is the primary regulator and maintainer of the immune system.

It also regulates the balance of the entire hormonal system. There is nothing that occurs in the body that is not in some major way regulated by the liver.

In contrast with the brain, however, the liver is not separated by a protective wall. It is right smack in the middle of all the nitty-gritty action.

Thus the liver is a vulnerable organ and needs all the help and care we can give it.

The fact that it is so vital to the maintenance of homeostasis, while at the same time so vulnerable to damage and dysfunction, is why I regard it as the most important organ in the body.

Let me put it another way. If you want to be healthy, do everything you can to help and protect your liver. As you read through the rest of this book, you will see that a huge part of my ten-step program involves therapies and lifestyle habits geared to helping the liver.

I have often thought that it is not accidental that the word liver starts with the word "live."

Just to review, the following basic components prevent the accumulation of toxins: increased energy production, water, fiber, sleep, movement, exercise, and nutrients that assist the liver and intestines. Along with these, we obviously should try to limit our exposure to toxic conditions and substances that can interfere with the elimination process by adding to the overall toxic burden. These substances include cigarette smoke, silver dental fillings, unnecessary pharmaceutical drugs, and inhaled or ingested environmental chemicals.

Part Two
Ten Secrets for Improving Your Energy

Secret No. 1
Drinking For Energy

Water has absolutely no nutritional value. Your body cannot produce energy from water. Nevertheless life would very quickly come to a halt without water.

You can go without eating for weeks, but you can't go without water for more than several days. The reason: 75 percent of your body is comprised of water. And every single aspect of biological functioning will quickly break down without enough water in your system.

A very simple home experiment can demonstrate this. Put a bit of baking soda and vitamin C powder into a glass. What happens? Absolutely nothing! Now add a little water and watch the powerful reaction that develops. In your body the same effect is at work.

Without adequate amounts of water every biochemical reaction, including those that are essential for the proper generation of energy, is compromised.

Take the brain as an example. It is an organ with a most complex biochemical reactivity. The speed at which these reactions occur is critical. Your information processing and thinking activity depend on it.

While most other organs in the body are made up of 75 percent water, the brain is said to consist of 85 percent. When the brain becomes even slightly dehydrated, your mental speed declines markedly. Greater levels of dehydration result in delirium and seizures.

Another critical aspect of water relates to detoxification. **Water is the only solvent that the body can use to rid itself of toxins.**

Some toxins, as we have discussed, are environmental. But the majority are formed inside the body as the waste products of normal metabolic function.

Without any water intake, these toxins would accumulate so rapidly that in most cases you would die within four or five days.

With a much less than optimal intake you wouldn't die, but you wouldn't be able to flush out the toxins fast enough. This would lead to chronic toxin accumulation, decreased organ function, and ultimately, disease.

Yet another vital function of water is the maintenance of body temperature. Your body's ability to cool itself depends on adequate water intake.

High fevers associated with acute illnesses, such as flu, are often the result of dehydration. And if you find you are intolerant of hot weather, the chances are that you are significantly dehydrated.

Think of water as the coolant you put in your car. If the level goes down too far, the engine overheats. It's the same with your body.

Few People Drink Enough

Despite its fundamental importance, it is amazing how few people actually drink enough water. In my clinic, I find that more than 30 percent of my healthy preventive medicine minded patients are chronically dehydrated. These patients all say they feel great, and have no symptoms, yet when I check their body water level they are clearly deficient.

And none of them ever respond positively when asked if they are thirsty. Although thirst is a pretty good indicator of acute dehydration, in chronic states of dehydration the body adjusts by retaining fluids, and so thirst doesn't occur.

Thirst, it turns out, is a poor indicator of adequate hydration. A 1998 article in the American Journal of Hospital Palliative Care dramatically points this out. The researchers reported that fluid depletion even in severely dehydrated dying patients resulted "in relatively benign symptoms," of which thirst was not a common one.

The bottom line here is that the lack of thirst doesn't mean you are not dehydrated. The only way to be sure you have adequate body water levels is to drink enough water to cause you to urinate every 3-4 hours.

When the body retains fluids in a state of dehydration, it is also retaining the toxins that those fluids were supposed to eliminate. This increases the level of toxins in your tissues, and sets the stage for chronic disease and premature aging.

Fereydoon Batmanghelidj, M.D., an expert on water and author of an excellent book entitled *"Your Body's Many Cries for Water,"* points out that the body has no water storage system to draw on in times of need. And those parts of the body that suffer most from a water shortage are those areas without a direct blood supply, particularly cartilage in the joints.

Painful joints, and even arthritic joints, can be a result of inadequate water intake, Batmanghelidj says.

This overlooked issue was cited in *"Preventing Arthritis,"* a book by pain specialist Ronald M. Lawrence, M.D., Ph.D. "I have indeed found that joint and pain problems are helped by water, and made worse when a patient is dehydrated or hardly drinks water at all," says Lawrence.

Cured With Water

Several years ago, a 72-year-old female patient made an appointment to see me and reported the following medical history:

Eight months earlier she had started to experience nausea. Her appetite gradually diminished and she began to lose weight. Her physician had prescribed various medications, including ulcers drugs, but nothing improved her condition.

Two months went by, and she began to develop a severe pain in her right hip. Her doctor knew that she had arthritic damage in this hip, and so concluded that the increase in pain meant that it was finally time for a hip replacement.

After several weeks of continued pain, she was admitted into the hospital and underwent surgery. Following the procedure her nausea worsened to the point that she vomited almost everything she ate. Because of her persistent post surgical pain she was prescribed more pain medication, and was ultimately placed on very high doses of strong narcotics. She was then discharged from the hospital.

However, she soon returned to the hospital with continued weight loss, nausea, and vomiting. She never complained of thirst. Scans, X-rays, and blood tests failed to reveal any abnormality, but she was obviously dehydrated and was treated for fluid replacement with intravenous salt water. Miraculously, her symptoms improved and after the third day she was allowed to go back home.

Two months later she came to my clinic complaining of a recurrence of all her symptoms: persistent joint pain, continued dependence on narcotic medication, and relentless nausea and vomiting.

The case stumped me. I tried a homeopathic approach, but was unable to make any inroads. It was not until I recommended she drink six ounces of water every hour that the situation changed.

Within several days, she completely turned around. The stomach symptoms disappeared. Her pain went away.

It turned out that the entire range of symptoms was due to dehydration. Had she been adequately hydrated from the beginning, I am sure she would have been able to avoid the surgery, and all the misery that she had experienced during those many months. Remarkably, during the entire time, she never once complained of thirst!

Water Purity

When I talk to my patients about water, I emphasize the importance of purity. Chlorine, fluoride, pesticide residuals, heavy metals, or hard minerals often contaminate common tap water. This means that the water carries toxins into your body, thus reducing its overall detoxification role.

Don't assume that your water source is clean. According to a 1993 statement from the Environmental Protection Agency, eight hundred and nineteen cities across the United States serve unacceptably elevated levels of lead in their water supplies to approximately thirty million customers.

Additionally, a quarter of the public water systems in the United States have been found in violation of federal standards for water purity. Several epidemics of infectious diseases have been traced to contaminated public and ground water.

I've been testing water for many years and rarely do I find any well or city water pure enough to generate optimum detoxifying effects in the body.

I recommend to my patients that they install a home purification unit. The key word here is "purified." Water labeled as spring water, mineral water, or drinking water is just not pure enough. Ideally, water should be purified using either a reverse osmosis or distillation method. My favorite method is reverse osmosis, because distillation units are more complex and expensive, and don't remove as many potentially harmful materials.

My Recommendations

❑ Drink at least one-half your weight in ounces of water per day. For example, if you weigh 180 pounds, drink a minimum of 90 ounces daily.

❑ On hot days or when exercising, twice that amount may be needed.

❑ Once your body is used to drinking this amount of water, you will begin to feel thirsty if you aren't getting enough. But as a rule don't rely on thirst to remind you to drink water.

❑ Remember that your lymphatic system has been collecting toxins and dumping them into your blood stream during the night. So it's a good habit to help the kidneys by drinking 16 to 32 ounces of water when you get up in the morning. This may take some getting used to, but it's worth it.

❑ Coffee, tea, juice, alcoholic drinks, and sodas are not water. Nor are they substitutes for water. In fact, they can actually intensify dehydration through their diuretic action.

Secret No. 2
Sleeping For Energy

Get plenty of rest. That's the age-old physician prescription for sickness. It's also a prescription for staying healthy. And to day, even in this modern age of medical marvels, it still holds true.

Yet I find that that the issue of adequate rest and sleep appears to be a major challenge for patients. I am constantly reminding them that rest is really important and not getting enough of it can be a major barrier to all their health and anti-aging goals. Often, my nagging doesn't sink in. Perhaps it's just too simple a concept.

And the attitude of catching up on lost sleep "when I have the time" just doesn't cut it. Without adequate sleep your M-Factor and your E.Q. will decrease. Sleep-deprivation shortens your life and increases the likelihood of a variety of diseases including cancer, obesity, and diabetes.

My observation over the years has been that those patients who sleep the best also feel the best. They are the healthiest.

According to a 1997 article in the *New York Times Magazine*, many sleep researchers believe that sleep deprivation is reaching "crisis proportions." This is a problem not just for serious insomniacs, but for the populace at large, the article said, and added: "People don't merely believe they're sleeping less; they are *in fact* sleeping less - perhaps as much as one and a half hours less each night than humans did at the beginning of the century - often because they choose to do so."

In a September 2000 report published in the British journal *Occupational and Environmental Medicine*, researchers in Australia and New Zealand found that sleep deprivation can have some of the same hazardous effects as alcohol intoxication. Getting less than six hours a night can affect coordination, reaction time and judgment, they said, posing "a very serious risk."

In 1999, Eve Van Cauter, a sleep researcher at the University of Chicago, reported in *Lancet* that lack of adequate sleep can create a pre-diabetic state in the body, which in turn can contribute to obesity. Van Cauter's suggestion came after a study in which six young men were allowed only four hours of sleep each night for a week. During the week the subjects were tested and found to have impaired glucose tolerance, essentially a pre-diabetic state.

The sleep-obesity connection is troubling from all angles. Obesity itself impairs sleep, thus setting the stage for a scary vicious cycle.

Van Cauter also points out that two very important hormones, growth hormone and leptin, are secreted primarily during the sleep hours. Leptin is a hormone that signals the body to stop eating.

"With the low leptin levels of sleep debt, your body will crave carbohydrate even though you've had enough calories," says Van Cauter.

Your Two-Phase Body

Your body runs basically on two twelve-hour phases. The time between 6 a.m. and 6 p.m. is called the "catabolic" phase. During this cycle your body is willing to do pretty much anything to keep you up and running. That means it is going to continually sacrifice Peter to pay Paul. Simplistically speaking, if your left leg needs something that your right leg has, your body will borrow it from the right leg and give it to the left. If your heart needs some raw material more urgently than your adrenal glands, the body will make sure that your heart gets it, and your adrenal glands will have to make due.

This process is called catabolism, and results in damage to certain tissues in order to keep others with a higher priority running efficiently.

But don't worry. Your body is quite smart.

Enter phase two: the "anabolic" cycle. This is the time when the body repairs all the damage and "borrowing" that went on during the catabolic phase. The body's repair hours are between 6 p.m. and 6 a.m.

We call the process "anabolism," and most of it transpires when we are sleeping (or should be). This is a key point. The body repairs damage through the medium of rather subtle energy fields that cannot be effective during the active part of the day. These fields organize the repair effort, and reach their maximum potential during sleep, particularly the deeper levels of sleep.

This is precisely why sleep is so important. **Without an adequate sleep period we are unable to fully repair the damage we create during the day.** A chronic lack of adequate sleep results in accelerated deterioration of the body, leading to premature aging. Sleep is even more important to those who exercise and lead very active lives.

If You Don't Snooze You Lose

As you already know, our stress oriented 24-7 lifestyles don't help us stay healthy. I love capitalism, but our daily decisions often reflect a greater desire to make sacrifices for money than for health. Getting enough sleep is a good example of this. In fact, many of us have actually adopted the attitude that "if you snooze you lose."

I often meet people who brag about how little sleep they need. "I can get by on only 4-5 hours of sleep and still exercise and have a fully productive day," they'll say. This macho attitude may impress some of their friends, but I see it more as an act of self-destruction. These individuals have no idea how negatively they are impacting their health.

Many people have gotten into the habit of going to bed late so they can watch the late evening news. They have been convinced by the news industry that the news actually changes from day to day, and so they don't want to end their day until they have been "brought up to date." Actually nothing could be further from the truth. I watch the news about once every 1-2 months, and I can honestly tell you that I miss absolutely nothing of any importance in between viewings. Similarly, the only thing I find interesting about the late night TV guest shows is why anyone would prefer them to a good book.

The Sandman Says....

❏ Take your sleep time seriously.

❏ Be sure to get eight hours of good solid uninterrupted sleep in a fully darkened room, ideally before the sun comes up. If you can't do this, blacken out your room or use eyeshades so that it is still dark even after the sun has risen.

❏ Avoid food or alcohol for three hours before bedtime.

❏ Lights left on in the room interfere with sleep. The production of melatonin, perhaps the single most important hormone for the immune system, occurs during sleep. It is immediately cut off by exposure to light. Decreased melatonin production is thought to be one of the factors leading to breast and prostate cancer.

❏ If you have to get up in the night for a trip to the bathroom, don't turn on the lights. Use a red colored night light. Red light does not seem to curtail melatonin production.

❏ If you routinely get up to urinate, restrict your fluids before bed time.

❏ Chronic insomnia is a serious health problem. If you have this problem, don't "solve" it by taking drugs. Instead, treat the problem. Studies show that sleeping medications interfere with the development of the deeper levels of sleep. Following my other "secrets" in this book, particularly exercise, adequate water intake, supplements, sunlight exposure, and breath meditation, can go a long way to relieving insomnia. Also limit your intake of all caffeinated drinks. If you are over 45, try .5 to 3 milligrams of melatonin before bedtime. Certain herbs, particularly valerian and chamomile, are especially helpful to induce sleep.

❏ Don't use anything electric on your bed, such as electric blankets or heating pads. These devices create an electrical field that significantly interferes with the anabolic repair process. Even when they are turned off, electric heating systems still maintain an electric field because they have transformers. That's right. Even when they're off, they're on! Just get rid of them, and get a good comforter. You'll like it better anyway.

Secret No. 3
Sunlight For Energy

Despite the fact that we couldn't possibly survive without it, and that we evolved without the benefit of sunscreen or sunglasses, the sun has become something of a medical scapegoat, virtu ally synonymous with skin cancer.

But it makes no sense at all to me to indict the sun for the rise in skin cancer, the most commonly occurring cancer in the United States. Or, as some experts have done, blame it on the hole in the ozone layer that lets in more of the sun's ultraviolet (UV) rays. The hole is restricted to the area over Australia and thereabouts, and fails to explain the dramatic increase in skin cancer *all over the world*.

Moreover, one study demonstrated a higher incidence of melanoma (a very serious type of skin cancer) among Australian *office workers* than among outside workers.

I believe we can attribute a good deal of the increase in skin cancer to the very same factors that have brought about an increase in *every* other type of cancer: *decreased energy production, toxicity, stress, and poor food choices.*

In 1982, a comprehensive report by the National Research Council on *Diet, Nutrition, and Cancer* concluded that much of the rising cancer rate in the U.S. was due to the typical American diet. And, according to the National Academy of Sciences, 60 percent of all cancers in women, and 40 percent of all cancers in men may be due to diet alone.

Smoking and passive exposure to cigarette smoke has also been linked to the increased incidence of all cancers, including skin cancer.

For sure, overexposure to the sun - and resultant sunburn - definitely increases the incidence of a type of common skin cancer called basal cell carcinoma. This is well documented. It is not known yet, however, whether similar over exposure is much of a factor in melanoma.

What is known is this, and sun worshipers should pay heed: sunburn, even slight sunburn, does cause premature aging of the skin, including wrinkles and pigmentation.

So it is advisable during the summer to limit exposure between 11 a.m. and 3 p.m., and don't let yourself become burned.

Am I telling you to stay out of the sun? No, far from it. Just be cautious.

There's no big secret about that. It's common sense.

My energy increasing secret involves the flip side of all this caution. By that I mean the essential and positive aspects of sunlight and just how valuable this primordial asset it is to your health. This is really an overlooked issue. I am more concerned about the health of people who don't get enough sunlight.

According to the late Dr. John Ott, an expert in the biological effects of light therapy, there is no doubt that too much UV is harmful. "But the fear of ultraviolet is causing people to overprotect themselves from sunlight to the point that they are creating a deficiency of a very essential life-supporting energy," he concluded.

Don't Become "Eclipsed"

Shut-ins, sun shunners, and office workers run the risk of sunlight deficiency. Your doctor may not tell you this but sunlight deficiency results in biological imbalances that will lower both your M-Factor and your E.Q. Moreover, it can cause decreased energy production, depression, anxiety, osteoporosis, hypothyroidism, insomnia, and immune suppression leading to both breast and prostate cancer.

Sunlight Deficiency = Energy Deficiency

Are you getting enough sunlight? The fact that sunlight is an important factor in energy production is well established. Many studies have shown a decrease in the basal metabolism of both animals and people when they do not receive enough sunlight. The decline in M-Factor commonly seen in everyone during the winter is a direct result of decreased sunlight exposure.

Sunlight deficiency is usually not an issue for those who live in the southern latitudes. Sunlight is readily available all year long.

However, for those in the north, it's a different story. In colder climates, the shorter days of winter and late fall can especially be a problem. Bundled up from head to toe, millions leave for work and return from work in the dark. And the weather keeps them inside during the day for weeks and even months without exposure to sunlight.

This single factor is undoubtedly what triggers flu epidemics during the cold months.

Well, you may be thinking, I work in a glass-encased office building and the light comes streaming through the glass. Sorry. That's not much help. Glass interferes with the absorption of certain spectrums of UV light that are critical to the function of the immune system. Exposure to sunlight through windows is better than none at all but it is of limited usefulness, and will not completely provide for your biological needs. You need the real thing - sans glass.

Sunlight exposure is also important for those who work under conventional florescent lights. They are deficient in certain spectrums. If possible, try to have full spectrum florescent lighting installed. If that's not an option, be sure to get out in the sunlight.

Our Healing Sun

In the late 1800s and early 1900s tuberculosis was a serious and widespread problem without an effective treatment. It was during this time that a Danish medical researcher named Niels Finsen developed a successful ultraviolet (UV) light treatment for an infectious skin disease called lupus vulgaris, for which there had been no cure.

Ultraviolet refers to the radiation that comes naturally from the sun. Some manmade lamps can also produce UV. For most of us, however, the sun is the primary source of UV. Finsen and his successors were able to demonstrate a remarkable 98 percent success rate simply by exposing affected areas of the body to UV light. He subsequently discovered something even more exciting. He had wondered whether the success of the treatment was due to a direct anti-bacterial effect of the light on the skin, or whether the results could be explained by the effect of the light on the immune system.

To determine this, he treated a number of patients with the disease by exposing only the *unaffected* parts of their skin to the light. He discovered that even when infected skin was not directly treated, the infection cleared up just as rapidly as it did in those in whom he directly treated the infected areas. **In other words, it was not the light itself that was killing the infection, but some internal physiological process that was stimulated by the light.**

For his breakthrough in demonstrating the healing power of light, Finsen was rewarded with the Nobel Prize in physiology and medicine in 1903. The award was given "in recognition of his contribution to the treatment of diseases, especially lupus vulgaris, with concentrated light radiation, whereby he has opened a new avenue for medical science."

What Finsen didn't know - but we know today, a century later - is that he was stimulating Langerhans cells in the skin. These cells are vital to immune system function. They are important antigen "presenting" cells, meaning that they communicate (that is, "present") the infection to other immune cells. This, in turn, initiates a proper immune response.

The Sun Doctor

Perhaps it is the effect of sunlight on the Langerhans cells that accounts for the most amazing of all stories regarding the use of sunlight to treat disease. Following Finsen's breakthrough research, a medical doctor named Auguste Rollier opened a "sun clinic" in the Swiss Alps, high above the cloud layer. **There, at "Le Chalet" as he called the place, he developed the therapeutic use of sunlight, along with rest, fresh air, exercise, and a balanced diet, into a powerful healing art form.**

This was an era before the advent of antibiotics, and Rollier documented many impressive cures for tuberculosis and other "incurable diseases."

His patients resided in hospital rooms, which had huge glass windows, and were oriented toward the sun. In addition, the rooms had balconies large enough to accommodate a bed. Patients, in beds or chairs, exposed themselves to the sun for about two or three hours a day in the summer, and three or four hours a day in the winter.

Rollier was convinced that sunlight, combined with excessive heat had negative effects on his patients, so he did not allow them out in the middle of the day during the warm summer months.

His success with tuberculosis and other infectious diseases was so significant that Rollier established some thirty-five "sun clinics" from 1903 to 1940, and at the height of his Alpine healing enterprise he was able to "treat" more than a thousand patients a day.

The controlled exposure to sunlight during periods lasting as much as eighteen months literally transformed sick, deformed children with spinal tuberculosis into healthy, energetic, fully functional youngsters with straight backs, who ended up being completely free of disease.

Rollier published extensively on the curative power of the sun, reporting not only miraculous cures of tuberculosis, but also success against abscesses and bone infections. His treatments were also effective for rickets, various anemias, and a variety of non-healing wounds.

For the record, not one case of basal cell carcinoma or melanoma was observed in any of the patients treated in these clinics. This is undoubtedly because along with adequate rest and a healthy diet, great attention was placed on being sure that the patients became gradually accustomed to the sun without getting sunburned.

Sunlight and Cancer

In recent times, the prevailing "sunlight-causes-cancer" bias has motivated researchers to focus on proving - in test tube experiments - that doses of UV light high enough to cause sunburn can damage the Langerhans cells. Most doctors are unfamiliar with the work of Finsen and Rollier, and have cited these test tube studies as "proof" that sunlight causes cancer.

In these studies, researchers invariably exposed various human cells in a test tube to extremely high doses of an unnatural spectrum of artificial light. I have not seen one study that actually used sunlight. Since these experimental conditions represent exposures both to light spectrums that just don't exist in nature and which are known to cause sunburn, it is not surprising that the exposed cells became damaged, and create changes consistent with cancer and damaged immune activity. Had the researchers paid much attention to the work of Finsen and Rollier, they would have learned that both of these doctors achieved their healing results without inducing sunburn.

Finsen and Rollier are classical examples of why we can't always translate isolated laboratory test tube findings to real life. Many times the results of such experiments bear little resemblance to what happens in vivo - that is, inside the body.

To further make my point, I'll cite a study conducted by dermatologists at the University of Turku in Finland that was published in the journal *Experimental Dermatology*. The researchers found that high doses of UV light could indeed damage Langerhans cells in a test tube. But when skin is exposed to UV, even high doses of it, the Langerhans cells are actually "up regulated," meaning they are stimulated. This study suggests that in reasonable doses, sunlight actually stimulates and enhances immune system function and efficiency, and helps to explain why Finsen and Rollier were able to cure the "incurable".

I am convinced that correct sunlight exposure and a healthy diet will prevent the very same skin cancers that some say are caused by the sun

The "Sunshine Vitamin"

Sunlight is the "rate-limiting" factor in the production of a very overlooked vitamin - vitamin D. The term rate-limiting means that if a necessary substance, in this case sunlight, is not available for a particular chemical reaction then the production of the end product suffers. Your skin tissue makes vitamin D, the degree of which depends on your exposure to sunlight. Not enough sunlight results in a deficiency of D. This is why vitamin D is known as the "sunshine vitamin."

The implications are immense. For one thing, vitamin D promotes the body's absorption of calcium, essential for the normal development of healthy teeth and bones. I'll be talking a lot more about calcium later on and, in "Secret No. 10" will discuss the overblown calcium-osteoporosis connection.

For now, let me just encourage you not to be misled into thinking that osteoporosis has anything to do with a dietary deficiency of calcium as is widely propagated. **Even in primitive cultures where the diet is often less than perfect, there is no evidence of a link between calcium deficiency and osteoporosis**. The reality is that if an individual's lifestyle includes a reasonable diet, along with sunlight and exercise, osteoporosis does not exist.

But office workers who go to and from work in the dark, without going outside during the day, and elderly folks who tend to stay inside during the colder months are definitely at risk.

One study published in 1979 in the *British Journal of Medicine* examined the vitamin D level of twenty-three seniors for a period of sixteen months. In July the subjects had normal vitamin D levels, but by November the levels had dropped by an average of 19 percent. By the following February, 65 percent! At this point almost one-half of the group had levels consistent with the development of osteoporosis! This is a startling demonstration of the powerful effect of sunlight deficiency.

Another common disorder associated with aging is gradual hearing loss due to otosclerosis, an abnormal growth of bone tissue in the inner ear. The growth prevents the ear from working properly. The hearing loss is sometimes accompanied by chronic ringing in the ears (tinnitus).

Otosclerosis is a multifactorial disease, that is, caused by a variety of factors. Among them: a deficiency of vitamin D. A 1985 study published in *Otolaryngology and Head and Neck Surgery* indicated for the first time that supplementation could help some patients as a low level of the vitamin may contribute to demineralization of bone tissue in the ear. Today, vitamin D is part of the medical treatment for otosclerosis. But it's my guess that if people got an adequate amount of sunlight during their lives there would be much less otosclerosis to begin with.

Vitamin D And Your Immune System

Vitamin D is deeply involved in proper immune system function, an overlooked fact that offers an additional explanation for the immune deficiency caused by inadequate sunlight exposure. Although the full mechanisms of this connection are unknown, a glimpse into the possibilities is provided by an article published in 1999 in *Cancer Research*. The article, written by Harvard Medical School researchers, concluded that the vitamin D deficiency *caused by elevated calcium intake* resulted in an increased incidence of advanced prostate cancer. The authors state, **"Our findings support increased fruit intake and avoidance of high calcium intake to reduce the risk of advanced prostate cancer."** Other studies show the same relationship with breast cancer.

Breast and prostate cancer aren't the only cancers associated with low vitamin D production. In an amazing nineteen-year study, published in the medical journal *Lancet* in 1985, researchers found that men with the lowest level of vitamin D (even though the level was still within the normal range) were more than twice as likely to develop colon cancer than individuals with the highest level.

A March 2002 article published in the medical journal *Cancer* examined cancer mortality in the United States as it relates to sunlight exposure. Deaths from a range of cancers of the reproductive and digestive systems were approximately *twice* as high in New England as in the southwest, despite a diet that varies little between regions.

The study, which examined 506 regions, found that the more ultraviolet B light people were exposed to the lower the cancer mortality. The study's author, Dr William Grant, says northern parts of the United States may be dark enough in winter that vitamin D synthesis shuts down completely. While the study focused on white Americans, the same geographical trend affects black Americans, whose overall cancer rates are significantly higher.

Darker skinned people require more sunlight to synthesize vitamin D. There are 13 malignancies that are apparently prevented by adequate sunlight exposure, mostly reproductive and digestive cancers. The strongest correlation is with breast, colon, prostate, and ovarian cancer. Other cancers apparently affected by sunlight include tumors of the bladder, uterus, esophagus, rectum, and stomach.

The Penetrating Power Of Sunlight

Since we don't run around in loincloths, you would probably think our clothes would block the powerful effects of sunlight.

Most people think that sunlight only affects the very outermost skin, but this is far from reality.

To see how deep light penetrates, William Campbell Douglas, M.D., a modern pioneer in the use of ultra-violet light therapy, offers a simple experiment in his fascinating book entitled, *"Into The Light."* Simply darken the room you're in and hold a flashlight under your hand. The light actually shines through the entire thickness of your hand.

How much stronger is sunlight!

Try the same experiment with some cloth material between your hand and the light, and you will find that the results are not all that different. The light still comes right through.

To quote Douglas: "It doesn't take a rocket scientist to figure out that if you can see the light illuminating the top of your hand then, obviously, the light has penetrated your hand."

Sunlight indeed can penetrate into the body even through clothing, causing an increase in energy production, increased vitamin D synthesis, and increased immune system function.

My Recommendations:

❑ Remember that too much of anything, including sunlight, can be harmful.

❑ The best time of day for sunbathing is during the morning hours.

❑ Start off your exposure to the sun gradually, and cover your face. Sunbathing should not include the face because it already gets plenty of exposure and excessive sun will cause wrinkles.

❑ Never expose your skin to an amount of sunlight that will create more than a barely perceptible reddening of the skin twenty-four hours later. If you are fair skinned, this may be no more than 10 minutes at first.

❑ Don't use sunscreens when you sunbathe. They interfere with the full spectrum of the light. Use them only in situations, such as in certain athletic activities, where cover protection is impractical, and where without sunscreen you will become burned.

❑ Wear a hat so that the thin, ultra-sensitive skin of your face, head, and neck is protected. The skin in these areas receive much more of the exposure than other parts of the body. Protecting them can minimize wrinkles, age spots, and blemishes that will make you look older than you really are.

❑ If you live in northern latitudes, take two or three cod liver oil capsules per day during the winter, just to ensure an adequate dietary intake of vitamin D.   If possible, try to get outside in the middle of the day for at least twenty minutes during this period of the year.

Secret No. 4
Eating For Energy

I recently read an anti-aging book that emphasized the importance of hormone replacement, supplements, and exercise. The entire discussion of food was limited to one paragraph that basically repeated the worn-out mantra of keep fat intake below 30 percent and cholesterol intake below 200 milligrams.

Giving food such short shrift is a great disservice to the reader.

Healthy eating is essential to a healthy liver, and all the hormones and exercise in the world will not make up for an unhealthy, unnatural diet.

Healthy, natural foods provide essential nutrients, fats, and proteins without which the body will be utterly unable to efficiently produce energy. Deficient diets will inevitably result in a significant decrease in both your M-factor and your E.Q.

The fact is that today's standard Western diet puts the liver under siege from a barrage of drugs, food additives, pesticides, artificial colors, antibiotics, radiation byproducts, and preservatives.

Simply limiting fat and cholesterol intake isn't enough...and doesn't relate to what eating healthy is all about.

I have great compassion for the poor consumer walking the aisles of his favorite supermarket. What confusion! What choices! The creative genius of Madison Avenue reaches out with cute product names, radiant packaging, claims of "fortified ingredients," and a lot of misinformation to garner the sale.

In this fashion, more man made "foods" have been created over the last fifty years than Nature has produced throughout evolution.

I put the word "foods" in quotes because the human liver and intestinal tract have never seen these "foods" before. "New and improved foods" inevitably mean unbalanced, manmade concoctions packed with synthetic oils and processed, fragmented nutrients, while lacking fiber, trace elements, nutrient balance, amino acids, healthy oils, and complex starches. **These patented creations have absolutely nothing to do with real food.**

Whether it's a "40-30-30 energy bar" or a pop tart, a much better description for these creations of food technology would be *industrial waste*. Even real foods like milk have been so industrialized that they are no longer obtainable in their natural, raw state.

Unless you go out of your way to learn about real food, most of the information you are exposed to about nutrition comes from the same people that make the junk.

Confused? Sure you are.

Fortunately, I have a simple rule that can eliminate the confusion.

Shallenberger's Rule For Food Selection

Don't Buy Anything With An Ingredients Label!!!!!!!!!

Another way of saying this is to avoid anything not made by Nature. If Nature made the food, the FDA has certified that it doesn't need an ingredients label. If Nature didn't make it, then it wasn't made for you and your liver.

Eat foods without added ingredients. That's a huge world of selection, in case you're worried. Your choices include beans, legumes, whole fruit, dairy, eggs, unprocessed oils, fresh vegetables, nuts, seeds, meats, poultry, fish, oats, quinoa, brown rice, and on and on.

A diet high in non-labeled foods will ultimately be the best one for you.

Forget about simple and complex carbohydrate, fat percentage, fiber percentage, vitamin content, etc., and just choose based on whether there's an ingredients label or not.

The Exception: When To Read The Label

There's a slight catch here in the simplicity of this concept. It's this: not all foods have been created - or at least grown and marketed - equally.

What I mean is that many natural foods including meats, fruits, and vegetables are being increasingly irradiated with X-rays, and then contaminated with dyes, additives, antibiotics, and hormones!

This is, in fact, a huge problem, especially for our kids. It's one thing to dose up an adult with hormones, but it's quite another to expose infants and young children to these substances.

Moreover, there is much evidence to suggest that the rampant infertility among young men and the menstrual disturbances, endometriosis, and obesity so common in young women originates largely from the estrogen contamination of milk, beef, eggs, and poultry. Fortunately, hormone-free foods are available if you look for them. Look for "Hormone Free" on the label.

As of this date the FDA has not required special labeling of foods irradiated with radioactive materials. This is a travesty. There is substantial scientific data indicating that irradiated foods contain molecules that are completely unnatural and hence foreign to our immune systems. The long-term effects of irradiated foods aren't known, and I recommend that they be avoided as much as possible. Unfortunately, manufacturers who are radiating foods will probably not disclose what they are doing until this is required by the FDA.

The Fiber Connection to Health

Humans are omnivores. We were designed to consume both animal and vegetable food sources. It not only doesn't make any sense to be a vegetarian, it is unnatural and downright unhealthy. Strict vegetarians, called "vegans", universally test out badly on Bio-Energy Testing™. They inevitably have lower M-Factors and EQ's, and they usually have unacceptably elevated C-Factors.

But neither is it healthy to be a 100 percent meat eater.

It's all about balance.

And it's also about fiber, which you can't get in animal protein. You have certainly heard much about fiber, and now you'll hear a little bit more.

Dietary fiber, also known as roughage, is the portion of plant food that human digestive enzymes cannot break down. It is most readily available in whole grains (not whole grain flour), seeds, nuts, whole fruits, beans and vegetables. Fiber absorbs moisture, increases in size, gives the muscles in the intestinal walls something to grip on, makes the stool softer, regulates the balance of intestinal bacteria, and acts as a natural laxative.

Fiber helps detoxify the liver. When the liver removes toxins from the blood, it excretes many of them into the intestines in the form of bile salts. Fiber, especially the "soluble" fiber that is found only in fruits and vegetables, acts like a sponge to absorb these toxic salts and escort them out of the body in your bowel movement.

That's why regular bowel movements are so important to health. **Without regularity, accumulated toxins build up in the intestines and the rest of the body**. These toxins are often a major cause of heartburn and intestinal diseases.

Much overlooked is the fact that the friendly bacteria in our intestines feed on fiber. These beneficial micro-organisms perform a wide array of services, including the elimination of harmful bacteria, and the production of important enzymes, acids and vitamins. Even more important, they contribute to the efficiency of the immune system. When they become depleted, your ability to fight off infections is affected.

Hundreds of studies have linked low fiber diets to virtually every disease. These include acne, heart disease, cancer, epilepsy, gall bladder disease, kidney stones, hypertension, infection, lupus, learning disabilities, diabetes, ulcers, and obesity.

There's not a lot more that can go wrong with you than that, so make sure you emphasize high fiber foods in your diet. That means whole fruit, vegetables, and legumes. In terms of carbohydrates those foods that best fill the bill are found among middle and low glycemic foods. These are listed in the "The Glycemic Index" in my Secret No. 9 on metabolic weight management.

When you refer to this index you will quickly notice that the least-desirable foods, the high glycemic foods, are the refined carbohydrate items, namely flour products and sugar. These fractured foods have very little or no fiber, and create a major problem with the hormones regulating blood sugar balance.

Filling your stomach with high glycemic foods is an invitation to weight gain and low energy, as well as bacterial imbalance in the intestines. Individuals who are overweight and/or have fatigue, or who have elevated triglycerides or cholesterol, definitely need to follow a diet that restricts high glycemic carbohydrates. In particular, they need to limit the intake of sweets and foods made from flour such as bread and pasta. And yes, even the so-called "whole grain flour" products test out just as bad as the white ones.

Please watch the sweets! Anything with added sugar should be considered as a "treat," and not real food.

One last word about flour and sweets. When you do indulge yourself, definitely avoid doing so on an empty stomach. The negative effects of these foods are maximized when eaten by themselves. Eat them only after you have already ingested some fat and protein, such as in the case of a dessert. That minimizes their impact on the physiology.

Fat: More Than Just Energy

Whenever I start discussing diet with patients, the first thing out of their mouths is that they are really trying to cut down on the fat.

What a great brainwash the food industry has accomplished! Almost everybody thinks of fat as something to be avoided like the plague. The majority of the population has been long convinced, and even "experts" buy into it, that for the sake of health we should invest our food dollars in industrially altered food that has had the fat removed.

"Fat's the enemy," we are repeatedly told. And, like the cavalry, the food manufacturers are riding to our rescue with low-fat and non-fat substitutes to protect our health and correct the mistakes of Nature.

I used to buy into this nonsense as well. Years ago I also believed that dietary fat raised blood fats and created atherosclerosis, hypertension, and heart disease. I was convinced that dietary fat was the cause of obesity. I even remember one expert who wrote that dietary fat caused diabetes.

I began putting all my patients on low-fat programs. Guess what happened?

Nothing!

Almost nobody lost weight. Heart disease and hypertension didn't improve, and my patients continued to complain of fatigue, depressed immunity, insomnia, and so forth.

Then I learned that I was being too flexible, that I was not sufficiently restricting fat.

"No more than 15 to 20 percent of your dietary calories should be in the form of fat," came the word from the experts. So, still convinced, I clamped down and recommended that my patients eat even less fat. Regardless of studies and what experts say, there is really no better litmus test than patient feedback. Patients live in the real world. Not in laboratory cages.

Physicians should always keep up on the literature, but when a study leads to recommendations that just don't work with your patients, it should be ignored, and something else should be tried.

Low Fat Diets = Low Energy

My patients did not improve on low fat diets. Moreover, they were beginning to resent me for putting them on a program that was extremely difficult to follow and did not taste good.

The lack of results and the negative reactions caused me to do a lot of re-thinking.

I was indeed "practicing" medicine by placing my patients on an abnormal diet. The human body did not evolve on a low fat diet. Anthropological studies overwhelmingly concur that the original human diet was filled with meat and fat. **Studies of the Eskimos and the Masai who literally eat virtually nothing but meat and fat revealed a complete absence of heart disease, hypertension, and diabetes**. It was only when they "modernized" and began eating flour and sugar that they developed these diseases.

I began thinking about the diets of patients when they first came to me. I asked myself how many obese patients ate a diet high in fat? I checked the dietary records.

The answer: None.

How many of my patients with heart disease actually ate a diet high in fat?

None.

How many of my patients with eating disorders gorged themselves on fat?

None.

Why not?

The answer came to me rather quickly when I finally asked the right question. People do not develop diseases or obesity from eating too much fat. It can't be done. You can't eat too much fat even if you try.

I once experimented on myself. I broiled a well-marbled steak, then covered it with butter. I quickly discovered that I was stuffed before I had even finished half of it.

Compared to carbohydrate, fat and protein sit very long in the stomach in order to be digested. So you feel full.

As I researched this further, I learned that fat induces the release of a hormone called cholecystokinin that causes the brain to rapidly register satiety. It turns out that it is literally impossible to overeat on a diet high in meat and fat. Blood sugar actually stabilizes, and many disorders of the stomach and bowels improve.

I've talked about fat as a basic energy food. But it is so much more. It is definitely something *not* to be avoided.

All our cell membranes are made from fat. And over half the energy our cells produce goes into maintaining the integrity of these membranes. Research has shown that the very first pathological findings, when cells become diseased or poisoned, occur in the membranes.

Think of the cell as an exclusive club. The cell membrane is like the front door. Nothing gets in or out without going through this door. It takes proper functioning of the membrane to allow entrance to all the vitamins, minerals, glucose, fat, and proteins needed as raw materials to fuel activity inside the cell.

And located on the membranes are receptor sites for hormones. This is where hormones, which are messenger proteins, transfer their regulatory commands to cells. Without healthy membranes the hormones cannot do their jobs.

Your nervous system and your brain are almost completely comprised of fats.

Fats also serve as the building blocks for the steroid hormones such as cortisol, DHEA, and all the sex hormones.

Fats make up prostaglandins, compounds that are intricately involved in the function of the immune system, the cardiovascular system, and the healing process after injury.

From this understanding, we can understand why Nature gave us fat to eat. And why fats should be appreciated and not avoided. Without an adequate supply of fat, we could not even begin to maintain our mental and physical health.

Not All Fats Are Created Equal

My last statement needs to be qualified. I should say, without an adequate supply of the right fats.

Nature indeed has given us fat to eat. So, too, has man. And it is with the man-made fats that the problems start.

Take one guess as to which fats lead to immune suppression, heart disease, diabetes, macular degeneration, arthritis, hormonal deficiencies, and premature aging.

Guess which fats the food industry has been pushing. Decades ago, food manufacturers encountered a problem transporting and storing processed "foods" because the fats in their products quickly became rancid. In order to make their merchandise more widely available the industry had to surmount the rancidity issue.

Food scientists provided the answer: technology known as "hydrogenation" and "partial hydrogenation". These methods alter naturally occurring fats in such a way that they do not become rancid. Moreover, these new fats are so foreign to Nature that even bacteria and insects can not survive on them.

The ideal commercial fat was created. A fat that could be stored for years without rancidity or attack from Nature's predators.

Man had "improved" the old-fashioned natural animal and vegetable fats, which, alas, become rancid if not refrigerated. Now we had margarine. It could sit on the counter top and thumb its nose at the oxygen in the air that causes rancidity.

Man could now have a cornucopia of new "foods" with enormous shelf life by using hydrogenated and partially hydrogenated fat technology in breads, mayonnaise, peanut butter, breakfast cereals, ad infinitum.

The only problem with the breakthrough is that these synthetic fats are alien to the body.

They can't perform all the healthy functions that fats are supposed to perform. Instead they actually interfere with the function of natural fats.

They don't maintain adequate cell membrane potentials. They adversely effect the cell membrane receptors that are basic to hormone function. They create imbalances in the body's inflammatory response, and, in fact, increase inflammation. They block the activity of the enzyme plasmin that dissolves platelet clots. This effect increases the risk of developing blood clots that can cause life threatening heart attacks.

Recent publications have also demonstrated that artificial fats actually damage the inner walls of the arteries, thus contributing to cardiovascular disease. Researchers have documented that the increased consumption of margarine exactly parallels the modern day epidemic of heart disease.

Other studies have shown that manmade fats change the composition of the cell membranes in the heart, and that these changes are associated with heart disease.

The bottom line: *Don't be concerned about how much fat you eat. Just be concerned about what fat you eat, and avoid hydrogenated and partially hydrogenated foods like the plague.*

High Fat and Low Fiber

What about medical reports showing an increase in cancer among people who eat high fat diets?

First, let me say that many of these studies are seriously flawed. Total caloric intake and incidence of obesity are almost never taken into account. The numbers of people monitored in these studies are relatively small and the supposed increase in cancer is modest at best. Moreover, there are many contradicting studies.

For example, breast cancer is often said to be strongly associated with excessive dietary fat. In a long-term study monitoring the health and habits of 90,000 nurses, some 601 cases of breast cancer developed. However, there was no evidence of any relationship to fat intake.

In another study, published in the Journal of the National Cancer Institute, researchers pointed out that while obesity and excess calorie intake have been implicated in cancer in both human and animal studies, fat intake per se has not. In this study, rats were exposed to a breast cancer-causing agent and then fed a diet high in fat but restricted in calories, or a diet low in fat but with a much higher level of calories in the form of carbohydrate. **Only 7 percent of the rats on the high fat diet developed breast cancer compared to 43 percent of those on the low fat, high calorie/carbohydrate diet.**

Unlike the supposed dietary fat connection, a review of the medical literature reveals many impressive studies linking deficiencies of fiber, vitamins, and other nutrients to cancer. I believe that any possible fat connection can be explained by the fact that diets high in fat often tend to be low in fiber.

It is not the high fat but rather the low fiber and deficient nutrient intake that presents a risk. Such deficiencies arise from diets lacking whole fruit, fresh vegetables, and legumes. So don't be concerned about eating too much fat, instead just make sure that your diet contains an abundance of whole fruit, veges, and legumes.

Protein: The Stuff You're Made Of

While fat and carbohydrate serve the body as sources of energy, protein forms the structural material of most of your body and is also involved in much of the biochemical business going on around the clock in your physiology. Your cells need enough protein, particularly animal protein, in order to make muscle tissue, produce hormones, enzymes, immunoglobulins, and brain neurotransmitters, and repair damaged organs.

Unfortunately, due to the popularity of vegetarian eating, many health conscious people have been led to believe that meat, eggs, and dairy are unhealthy for them. Additionally, since Nature designed that meat and fat travel together, the low fat frenzy has also resulted in a decrease in protein intake.

An insufficient intake of high-quality dietary protein results in chronic infections, low blood sugar, hormonal deficiencies, attention deficit syndrome, osteoporosis, arthritis, immune deficiencies, and virtually every other degenerative disease associated with aging.

The preferred protein sources are eggs, beans, tofu, dairy, and meats. Since no single source of protein is totally adequate, make sure you eat a variety of meats and beans. Also, make sure that you eat a significant amount of protein with virtually every meal. And keep in mind that the more you exercise or exert yourself, the more protein you will need.

Eat Less As You Get Older

As we age, we require fewer calories. This is true even if our lifestyle and exercise level remain in a youthful fast lane. For example, a 60-year-old man with the exact same activity level of a 40-year-old requires fewer calories to fulfill his energy needs.

So a major golden rule of eating as we age is to only eat as much as we need.

And a second rule is to lower the percentage of calories we get from high glycemic carbohydrates.

Dietary carbohydrate content for most 20 or 30 year olds should be around 50 to 60 percent of the total calories. However, as we approach 50 we should reduce the intake of high glycemic carbs so that total dietary carbohydrate content ends up being in the area of 40-45 percent.

Since every human system is unique, some persons will need to adhere to these guidelines more than others.

You will know how well your diet is working by how you feel. Are you strong, energetic, and "clean?" That is, free of excess toxins?

Thanks to Bio-Energy Testing™, we can precisely determine the answers by examining your C-Factor, your M-Factor, and your E.Q.

The Power Of Fasting

As long as you are healthy you can help keep yourself that way with regular short fasts. Animal studies have conclusively proven that fasting can significantly extend life span.

Basically anytime you don't eat for two or three hours, your body begins to go into a fasting mode. Fasting, and even just skipping meals, has been shown to elevate growth hormone levels by as much as 400 percent. When you read my Secret No. 8 you will learn why this is a most desirable result.

Regular short fasting is also a superior way to detoxify the body. Many toxins, particularly heavy metals, organic acids, and substances known as advanced glycosylated end products (AGEs), become lodged in the interstitial space between cells. This is not just a domain of empty space, but an active and systemic-wide production field where collagen is formed. Collagen is major protein molecule that makes up the basic substance of tissues, holding our bones, skin, blood vessels, and joints together.

The presence of toxins in this area interferes with the function of collagen. This undesirable process results in what is referred to as "cross-linking." When collagen becomes cross-linked, it loses its elasticity and becomes hard and brittle. You very vividly see the effects of cross-linking in the wrinkled skin of older persons.

Cross-linking is more than just skin deep. Its nasty effects are all over, in virtually every tissue. Cross linking is what causes old arteries to be stiff and fragile, leading to high blood pressure, heart disease, and strokes.

Fasting helps cleanse the body of many of the toxic molecules that contribute to cross-linking. Exercise and saunas also have the same effect, but fasting is very special in its own way.

I'm not an advocate of extended fasting. That's because there is too much protein loss from the body. Moreover, I believe that the same

How To Do A 36-Hour Fast

First Evening

❑ Finish supper by 7 p.m. Take 3 pancreas enzyme capsules at bedtime, no sooner than 10 p.m.

Next Day

❑ During the day drink at least 2 quarts of water. Each quart should containing the juice of 1 lemon and a tablespoon of either honey, molasses, or maple syrup.

❑ Morning: Take 3 pancreas enzyme capsules along with 1 quart of plain water immediately after you rise.

A half to one hour later, take 2 scoops of QuickStart™ mixed in a glass of plain water. With it take 2 cayenne capsules and 2 acidophilus capsules.

❑ Noon: Take 2 cayenne capsules.

❑ Afternoon (3 to 5 p.m.): Take 3 pancreas enzyme capsules.

❑ At suppertime: Take 2 scoops of QuickStart™ mixed in a glass of plain water. Take 2 cayenne capsules and 2 acidophilus capsules with it.

❑ At bedtime: 3 pancreas enzyme capsules.

benefits reaped from long fasts can also be achieved by a series of regular short fasts.

I personally try to get in one or two short (thirty-six hour) fasts every month and have recommended this to my patients as well. More frequent fasting is a particularly good idea for individuals with diabetes, hypertension, or any degenerative disease process. But those with medical conditions should only fast under the guidance of an experienced health professional.

The 36-hour-fast I describe below represents a very do-able clean up act. Basically, it involves not eating after 7 p.m. on one day, skipping food all the next day, and then breaking the fast the following morning.

During the fast you'll be using some supplements that I highly recommend. They include QuickStart™, a special high-fiber nutritional formula that I developed (I describe it in detail in the next chapter).

In addition you'll be drinking at least two quarts of water throughout the fasting day that is "spiked" with the juice of a lemon and honey, molasses, or maple syrup to keep your blood sugar steady.   It's very

Second Day

❑ Morning: Take 3 pancreas enzyme capsules along with 1 quart of water immediately after you rise.

A half to one hour later, take 2 scoops of QuickStart™ mixed in a glass of plain water, along with 2 cayenne capsules and 2 acidophilus capsules.

During the rest of the morning eat 1 piece of whole fruit and drink the honey/lemon water mixture if desired.

❑ Lunch: Break the fast with a salad   .

Note

The exact doses of each of the pancreas, acidophilus, and cayenne capsules are not that important. Your local health food store can help you here.

Whenever you take the pancreas enzyme capsules, do not take the honey/lemon water mixture for 30 minutes before or after to avoid diluting the detoxifying effect of the supplement.

You may also drink up to 8 ounces of coffee or 8 ounces of green tea per day if desired. Drink as much herbal tea as you like.

If you take hormones or medication, continue as normal.

simple. And very effective. The time goes by very quickly. Just be sure to select fasting times that are comfortable for you and can fit into your schedule of activities.

If the fast is still too long for you, just remember that skipping a meal here and there will also help detoxify you.

The benefits of fasting also extend to the emotional area. Even though it doesn't seem to make a lot of sense, virtually all of us depend to some degree on regular meals to confirm a sense of safety and security. **For these reasons, it is very common to confront uncomfortable feelings such as boredom, anger, insecurity, guilt, anxiety, sadness, and low self esteem when going on a fast.** Sometimes these emotions can be quite intense. These feelings indicate our emotional connections with eating, and for many people this revelation will become quite an eye opener.

Many of us either eat too much, or eat foods that we know are poor choices, simply to abate current emotions. Fasting presents a wonderful opportunity to examine just how much these suppressed emotions may be running our lives without us really realizing it. And for those who like personal insights, a fast offers impetus to deal with emotions in a healthy way, rather than continuing to suppress them under a barrage of chocolate, chips, crackers, or other goodies.

Fasting can also instill a sense of gratitude for living in a country where hunger is relatively rare. Gratefulness is surely one of the healthiest anti-aging emotions.

My Diet

Patients always ask me how I eat. So, in case you too are curious, here's the kind of diet I generally follow.

For breakfast I down a "smoothie" containing QuickStart™ (the super supplement I describe in the next chapter), a carrot, a half of an apple, a half-teaspoon of turmeric, a couple of thin slices of ginger, and a tablespoon of flax oil. I blend it together in enough water to make the consistency just right. For me that means about 10 ounces of water.

This combination drink is so totally balanced in nutrients, carbohydrate, protein, and fat that it is often all I eat in the morning. If I happen to get hungry later on in the morning I will munch on whole fruit such as cherries, oranges, apples, apricots, peaches, berries, pears, or plums. I tend to avoid melons, pineapples, bananas, and mangos because they are high glycemic foods (see the glycemic index list on page 167).

On the mornings I plan a long bike ride or a weight lifting workout, I will add some additional protein in the form of eggs or meat.

For lunch I have one of several options: 1) a salad with ranch house dressing, cheese and meat; 2) a bowl of soup; 3) a meat sandwich; or 4) a bean, cheese, and meat burrito.

For supper I eat a salad, fresh vegetables, some form of meat or tofu, and perhaps additional beans.

I don't usually snack or eat sweets.

My goal is to eat at least three servings of different vegetables a day, and at least one fresh salad. Since every vegetable and fruit has its own unique nutrient content, I make sure I eat a variety.

I try to keep the bread, rice, and pasta to a minimum.

I am not concerned about eating too much fat or protein, and I strictly avoid non-fat or reduced fat foods.

I eat very slowly, thoroughly chewing my food (which is very impor tant for good digestion), and am usually the last one at the table to fin- ish.

I avoid overeating.

Mornings are the most important time of the day from the angle of detoxification. That's the time to emphasize high nutrient, fiber, and liquid intake. That's why I start off my days with a quart of water and a QuickStart™ smoothie.

My Recommendations:

❑ As much as possible, avoid manmade foods, particularly sweets and non-fat or reduced fat foods.

❑ Limit your intake to 4-8 ounces of organic coffee a day. Too much coffee is hard on the liver, and contributes to allergies and various digestive tract disorders. Moreover, too much java cre- ates an acid condition in the tissues and acts as a diuretic. This combination contributes to osteoporosis because when the level of acidity rises in the body, the system responds by pulling cal- cium out of bone tissue to buffer the acid.

If you enjoy the stimulant effect of coffee, you might want to give green tea a try. Not only is it a strong stimulant, but it also has anti-cancer properties.

❑ For these same reasons, limit alcohol to one drink a day. In small amounts, alcohol can also have a beneficial stimulatory effect on the liver like coffee. But in excess, as is universally known, alcohol can cause many problems.

❏ Modern, mass-production milk has been ruined by the homogenization and pasteurization processes. Even in small amounts it often triggers allergies. In larger amounts, it often causes bowel and liver problems. So try to avoid milk.

Yes, milk contains a lot of calcium, but it has no fiber. Actually you can get more calcium per gram of weight from spinach and other vegetables than from milk.

Children do not need milk at all. Children who don't drink milk have bones just as strong as their milk-drinking friends, and they avoid the common problems associated with milk ingestion.

Dr. Frank Orski, director of the Department of Pediatrics at Johns Hopkins Hospital, has pointed out that milk contributes to diarrhea, constipation, anemia, skin rashes, ear infections, and hyperactivity in children.

❏ Avoid sodas, sugar, breakfast cereals, sweets, fast food, and junk food.

❏ When you do eat sweets, eat them in the form of a dessert, that is, after a meal. Avoid sweets, cookies, and cakes on an empty stomach. By eating them after a meal you dilute their sugar content with the other foods already in your stomach.

❏ Artificial sweeteners are OK two or three times a week.

❏ Use Pam, lecithin, olive oil, or butter when you cook. Avoid deep fried foods. Learn to lightly sauté foods in a little olive oil or butter.

❏ Never use margarine, shortening, hydrogenated or partially hydrogenated oils, or the "foods" that contain them.

❏ Forget fruit juice. It is not a health food. Drink juice only sparingly, as a treat. Why? It has no fiber, and is high in sugar. Did you know that a glass of most fruit juices contains as much sugar as a cola?

❏ Keep your breakfasts and lunches light, and make supper the biggest meal of the day. There may be some exceptions to this rule in persons who have very physical jobs.

❏ Avoid going to sleep for at least three hours after supper. This means eating supper early, say around 6:00 p.m. Three hours is enough time for your body to digest the meal. If you are tired before that time, lie down and rest. But try not to fall asleep.

You cannot fully digest your foods while you sleep, and this will ultimately lead to increased toxicity and weight gain.

❑ Be consciously grateful for the blessing of good food you have.

❑ Chew your food well. Eat slowly. And enjoy what you eat.

❑ **My favorite recommendation: Feel free to break all the above rules periodically**. It's how you eat over the long-term that counts, not the transgressions you commit now and then. A healthy body can handle a toxic situation periodically, and besides it gives you something different to look forward to!

Secret No. 5
Supplements For Energy

It may seem like a fairy tale in this day and age, but once upon a time (and not so very long ago), taking vitamin and mineral supplements was quite a controversial issue for doctors. The position of the American Medical Association and many physicians emphasized the adequacy of a so-called "balanced diet." This was enough, it was believed, to provide all the nutritional requirements for the average Joe or Jane. In this mindset, many physicians argued that supplements could actually be dangerous, even though there was absolutely no evidence of medical injury from the proper use of supplements.

In recent years, the tide of opinion has turned significantly. The decade of the 1990s witnessed a huge wave of worldwide scientific validation for the use of supplements, ranging from vitamins and minerals to the most esoteric of rainforest herbs. Moreover, mounting consumer and patient interest has forced many doctors to rethink their attitude and modify an anti-supplement bias.

In addition, it has been widely recognized that large numbers of people don't eat a healthy, balanced diet. They eat imbalanced diets heavy in processed, convenience foods that *guarantee* nutrient deficiencies leading to health problems.

Today, physicians are routinely exposed to positive articles on the beneficial aspects of proper nutritional supplementation in leading medical publications, including the Journal of the American Medical Association. This development represents a 180-degree reversal of past policies.

We now see a plethora of articles citing all the many benefits of supplements such as:

❑   How B6, folic acid, and B12 help prevent heart disease.

❑   How oral magnesium tablets prevent fatal cardiac arrhythmias.

❑   How chromium supplementation aids diabetes.

❑   How vitamins C, E, and A, and the mineral selenium combat the development of cancer.

❏ How a simple extract of rice bran causes cancer cells to revert back into normal cells.

❏ How coenzyme Q10 rescues ailing hearts and also protects against the dangerous side effects of cholesterol lowering medication.

Keeping up with the nutritional research is almost a full time job. The information is torrential.

The question is no longer: "Should I be taking supplements?"

The question now is: "Which are the most important supplements for me and at what dosage?"

Proper, effective supplementation is really an individual matter. The concept of taking supplements according to RDAs - recommended daily averages of nutrients - is illogical. That's because we are all individuals with specific needs, conditions, and unique bodies.

Precise nutritional needs can only be determined using some fairly sophisticated testing, along with a detailed history and physical examination. Nonetheless, there is still much that can be said in a general way about taking supplements.

Principals of Supplementation

By providing and insuring optimal levels of all the nutrients that are so vital for the production of energy, proper supplementation can be pivotal in optimizing your metabolism and energy.

I have been testing the biochemical and nutritional patterns of my patients for over twenty years. This experience has taught me some important general principles regarding nutritional supplementation.

❏ Principal No. 1

Vitamin and mineral pills *don't work* unless they supplement a good diet. **Taking supplements while on a fast food, high glycemic, low fiber diet is a complete waste of time and money.**

Surprised? Don't be.

Supplementing a poor diet is like building an otherwise well constructed house on quicksand. It would be impossible for you to get all the nutrition you need even if you took a hundred supplements three times a day. Every nutrient requires a multiplicity of other nutrients to be present in order for it to exert its own particular effect. Only a non-toxic, nutrient dense, high fiber, high protein diet, such as the type I discussed in the previous chapter can guarantee this.

❑ Principal No. 2

Supplements should be taken in a balanced way.

Typically, people read a magazine article extolling the virtues of a "new, super nutrient." Then they rush out, buy the supplement, and start taking it.

Forgotten in this willy-nilly approach is that *additional supplementation is often required* to preserve the balance needed to support and bring out the effect of the "super nutrient."

Always remember that vitamins and minerals work together as a team. For instance, vitamin E, the amino acid cysteine, and selenium work together to form glutathione peroxidase, a star antioxidant enzyme produced in the body.

Your supplementation program should always reflect respect for balance and synergism. You do best with a broad range of nutrients, not just popping the "supplement of the month."

❑ Principal No. 3

The issue of dosage is often abused.

When you increase the dose of one nutrient you may need to increase the doses of some or all of the others, or else you invite imbalance.

The principle is this: it is best to use relatively small doses of many nutrients rather than large doses of any one nutrient.

This is extremely important.

This approach is particularly valuable when it involves antioxidant nutrients such as vitamin C.

While in the 1970's the so called medical and nutritional experts of the day declared it to be "unproven," today almost everybody is aware that a reduction in the antioxidant defense systems leads to cancer, AIDS, heart disease, and virtually every other degenerative disease known to medical science. This has contributed to the idea that the more "antioxidant" nutrients one takes, the more likely it is that antioxidant defense systems will be enhanced.

But is this true? Is it possible to take too much of an antioxidant and minimize its effect? Greater minds than mine have advocated routine megadoses of antioxidants, especially vitamin C, as a way to improve antioxidant defense mechanisms, but are they right?

I first started to consider this question in earnest after reading an article published in 1995 in the *International Journal of Biochemical*

Cell Biology. The article compared megadoses, typical supplemental doses, and RDA doses of vitamin E, and reached the following conclusion: "Further increases in vitamin E to megadose levels did not provide additional protection from oxidative stress." The term oxidative stress refers to damage created by free radicals, molecular fragments that spawn biochemical destruction and disease in the body.

In another study on vitamin C, it was also shown that megadoses are no more effective at immune stimulation than more conservative doses.

In these two studies, megadoses were not helpful, nor did they produce any negative effects.

However, in a 1983 article published in the Italian journal *Acta Vitaminologica et Enzymologica*, entitled "Effect of dietary coconut oil and casein and megadoses of vitamin A or C on tissue lipid peroxidation and hemolysis in vitamin E deficiency," researchers claimed that *megadoses* of vitamins C and A both caused an *increased* destruction of red blood cells secondary to oxidative damage.

In another study, an article entitled, "High Dose Vitamin C Decreases Liver Detoxification," the author asserted that "megadoses of vitamin C diminish the availability of cysteine," and thus render the liver more susceptible to oxidative damage! Cysteine, an amino acid, is a precursor to glutathione, a primary antioxidant and detoxifying protein in the liver.

These reports prompted me to conduct a small experiment in my clinic. I divided a group of volunteer patients in half according to whether they took megadoses of vitamin C or more moderate amounts. I then infused an intravenous solution that would create significant oxidative stress on their blood.

Blood samples were then taken and analyzed for the effects of oxidation. **The analysis showed that the antioxidant buffering capacity of those on moderate doses of vitamin C was significantly greater than those taking megadoses.**

I also discovered that the strongest antioxidant responses appeared to be those individuals who regularly engaged in aerobic excise.

The bottom line is that this research has led me to conclude that mega antioxidant supplementation is not required as a routine preventive measure. Such megadosing may actually decrease the body's ability to defend itself against oxidative stress. So don't megadose on your own. It is really a therapeutic concept that requires the guidance of a nutritionally savvy physician.

My Super Immune QuickStart™

In the previous chapter I introduced you to QuickStart™ a nutritional supplement that I developed and recommend to my patients. Throughout this book I will refer to it many times, so at this point I would like to go into greater detail, and tell you why I so vigorously recommend it.

I have put a lot of thought and 25 years of patient experience into the formulation of this unique blend of nutrients, herbs, and amino acids. While it was never meant to be a substitution for a healthy diet, I believe that the spectrum and doses of QuickStart™ reflect the current state of the art in medical and nutritional science.

I first began to make QuickStart™ more than 10 years ago for my own patients, long before it was commercially available. The results and feedback from patients has been so gratifying that in 2000 I decided to make it available to everyone.

I did not write this book to sell QuickStart™. I created the formula long before I wrote this book, to fill a vacuum. I wanted to save my patients the money and time required to take all of the ingredients separately. And there just wasn't anything in the marketplace that met my criteria.

I don't really care if you buy QuickStart™, or simply take all the ingredients found in it in a separate form. In fact, in case you want to do that, I have included in the appendix all the ingredients along with their doses. If you decide to take a substitute, that's OK, too. As long as you and your physician are happy, I'm happy. That having been said, here's the commercial.

QuickStart™ comes blended as an extremely fine powder. I tell patients to use it as part of a "power breakfast" smoothie that literally gives them a rocket launch boost off each morning.

It makes a delicious "one stop" therapeutic formula that provides all the supplementary nutritional and immune enhancement that most people will need. It is also designed to powerfully assist the detoxifying activity of the liver.

I haven't performed any double-blind clinical studies to demonstrate that QuickStart™ is any better than other herbal/nutrient mixtures. I just know it gets the results I am looking for and my patients are looking for.

The reason for its many gratifying effects is because the QuickStart™ formula works on so many basic levels. It is formulated to do the following:

❑ Enhance immunity

❑ Alkalinize tissues

❑ Improve circulation

❑ Stabilize the appetite

❑ Maximize liver function and detoxification

❑ Provide complete nutritional and anti-oxidant protection

❑ Remove heavy metals

❑ Increase energy production.

As you can probably guess, I would not design a supplement formula that doesn't specifically focus on providing *all* the various nutrients that your liver needs to keep your body maximally detoxified.

It is important to mention that QuickStart™ does not contain meaningless doses of many nutrients just to make the label look good. Every ingredient is tried and true, and is added in its *full therapeutic dose*.

I don't just recommend QuickStart™ to patients. I take it every day myself, and my whole family takes it as well. My patients tell me they wouldn't miss it for anything. It's a fabulous way to start the day.

A Dozen Reasons To Take QuickStart™

One

It provides both preventive and therapeutic benefits.

Two

It's effective, easy, and convenient. It comes as a fine powder that ensures maximum absorption, even for individuals with less than perfect digestive systems.

Much of the vitamin content of pills is ruined in the manufacturing process. Moreover, because of the complex nature of the digestive tract, the use of capsules and tablets are inferior ways of delivering nutrients. Pills often do not adequately break down, which means that much of their content is not absorbed.

It would require over 60 large-sized capsules to pack the same amount of nutrients found in a regular dose of QuickStart™. Few people will take that many pills for very long.

The formula has been carefully formulated and scientifically manufactured so that each vitamin, mineral, and herb is present and delivered in the most effective form.

Other supplements, if needed for a specific therapeutic reason, can be easily added to the mix.

Three

The formula tastes great. It mixes quickly and easily with water as a breakfast drink. Compared to pills, this is a much more natural and less complicated way to take nutrients.

Four

It's much more affordable than the many bottles of pills that would be needed to obtain similar protection. Recently I referred to the catalog of a major supplement retailer to determine the cost of ingredients in a one-month supply of QuickStart™ if the same ingredients were purchased separately. I calculated a total of $163. Since QuickStart™ sells for $58, that represents a difference of more than $100 per month.

Five

The formula satisfies the appetite and is thus beneficial as an aid for weight control (more about this in my Secret No. 9). The contents are low in carbohydrate and high in energy-boosting ingredients. It is suitable for all diets.

Six

QuickStart™ detoxifies the liver, and restores and maintains optimal bowel function.

Seven

It contains extra chromium - a full 1200 micrograms per serving - necessary for protection against blood sugar disorders in a society where high carbohydrate diets are contributing to rampant diabetes.

Eight

It contains a full therapeutic dose of astragalus, a superb Chinese herb that enhances immune cell effectiveness and antibody production, as well as inhibiting suppression of immune function by tumors.

Nine

It contains *therapeutic doses* of saw palmetto and soy isolates, shown to help prevent prostate and breast disease, regulate both male and female hormones, and enhance immunity.

Ten

A therapeutic level of ginkgo biloba helps inhibit platelet aggregation and adhesion, and decrease fibrinogen and plasma thickness. Translated from medicalese, this means a desirable blood-thinning activity. I believe gingko is much more effective in this regard than is aspirin, and has none of the dangers. Ginkgo also helps protect cell membranes, and quench free radicals. And, as is well known, it also improves blood circulation in the brain.

Eleven

QuickStart™ features a base of microfiltered, undenatured whey protein isolates. This material is rich in antibodies, lactoferrin, and glycomacropeptide (GMP). Lactoferrin binds free iron in the body, thereby reducing iron-induced free radical production. GMP stimulates the release of cholecystokinin, a potent hormone that signals satiety to the appetite control centers in the brain.

Twelve

The formula also benefits the heart and contains potent nutritional elements known to reduce the risk of cardiovascular disease. The unique combination of phytosterols, soluble fiber, niacin, B6, folic acid, B12, chromium, and antioxidants improves insulin sensitivity, lowers LDL cholesterol, triglycerides, and homocysteine levels.

A complete list of all the nutrients and their doses can be found in appendix B.

How to Order QuickStart™

QuickStart™can be obtained through the mail by calling 1-866-377-0610, or on the Internet by going to www.bursting-with-energy.com

Directions for Taking QuickStart™

I recommend taking QuickStart™ as a breakfast replacement. It is formulated to duplicate the composition of a perfect food.

Start with a half a scoop or less. The formula is quite strong and may take a few days for your body to get used to it.

Add one tablespoon of flax oil. This is very important!

Most of my patients add extras such as carrots or fruit. I personally add a carrot, half an apple, turmeric, and fresh ginger, but you can make it up anyway you want. Then add water and ice according to your preference, and blend it in a blender.

When traveling, just shake it up in a container with some ice water. Don't bother with the flax oil on the road because it requires refrigeration.

After you've grown adjusted to a starting dose of QuickStart™, gradually increase the daily dose to the recommended two scoops.

When you first start taking the formula you may experience a warm, prickly feeling on your neck and face. Don't be alarmed. This is just a cleansing reaction from the niacin. It will gradually disappear as you continue the program.

Think of QuickStart™ as your breakfast. It is an extremely good way to create a high energy level all day long.

My Three Month Rule

Every cell in your body except nerve and brain cells reproduce themselves within three months. This means that four times a year you get to have a practically brand new body! If these new cells are bathed in all the nutrients found in QuickStart™, guess what? They will be healthier than their predecessors. This rejuvenation phenomenon will continue until eventually you will feel as good as you've ever felt. Once you reach that optimum level of health and vitality continue to take one to two scoops every morning for maintenance.

My Recommendations:

❑ Keep it simple. Start off each day with a smoothie including two scoops of QuickStart™ and a tablespoon of flax oil.

❑ For individuals over fifty, take an additional 30 milligrams of co-enzyme Q10 and 100 milligrams of alpha lipoic acid.

Secret No. 6
Exercising For Energy

Few things perhaps are more misunderstood than exercise. In this country we have the concept completely backwards. Let me explain: On the one hand, we are almost obsessed with making sure that our kids get plenty of it. We make sure they have regular physical education classes. And if you've had children in the school system you know that getting them excused from P.E. usually requires something akin to a letter from the Pope. We go to great expense making sure that schools offer a large and diverse sports program, and enthusiastically encourage participation.

The irony in all this is that while exercise is obviously good for everyone, the primary needs of the under 35 crew are good nutrition and adequate rest. Exercise per se is not all that important.

However, somewhere around the age of thirty-five, our physiology starts to change in significant ways. And then, because of these changes, exercise begins to become less optional and more compulsory.

As we grow older our muscle mass steadily decreases and the metabolism levels off and begins to decline. This decrease in the metabolic rate is the single most influential factor in the genesis of the diseases and infirmities associated with aging. Bio-Energy Testing™ can detect the extent of this decline by a decreased M-Factor.

Exercise can effectively counter much of the age-associated decrease in the metabolic rate, and in the process strengthen the immune system, improve cardiovascular function, increase your E.Q., and slow down the rate at which you biologically age.

But go into a health club and what do you see?

Not many over 60-year-olds.

Mostly you see the younger set, while the majority of the older generation is home actively pursuing some version of couch behavior. The older folks have been told, "You need to take it easy. You're too old for that stuff."

The truth is just the opposite. They're too old *not* to do that stuff.

This is what I mean when I say that our society has it backwards when it comes to exercise. Exercising is a luxury for the young, but an absolute necessity for the old. Those of us who want to delay the aging process, and function at a much younger level, need to understand that *regular* exercise is *essential*.

Exercise Cuts Your Disease Rate

"A man falls into ill health as a result of not caring for exercise."

- Aristotle

Many gerontologists (medical experts specializing in treating older people) regard exercise as perhaps the closest thing to an anti-aging pill. They believe that a regular program of physical activity can go far in slowing or reversing many of the physiologic changes and illnesses associated with aging, and thus help restore youthful vitality.

Exercise as a "longevity elixir" has been the focus of an on-going world-famous study conducted by Stanford researcher Ralph Paffenbarger, Jr., M.D. With updates published over the years in leading medical journals, the study tracks exercise habits and longevity among more than 17,000 Harvard alumni. In a 1986 report for the *New England Journal of Medicine*, Paffenbarger revealed that his findings show that "For each hour of physical activity, you can expect to live that hour over - and live one or two more hours to boot."

And here's more evidence:

❑ According to Dr. Ken Cooper, M.D., of the Cooper Institute of Aerobic Research, there are 40 percent fewer heart attacks among women who exercise and 60 percent fewer among exercising males. In another study, he determined that individuals in the lowest 20 percent bracket of cardiovascular fitness had a death rate three times higher than the most fit group. The study also indicated that men who started exercise, even after the age of sixty, increase their life expectancy.

❑ Among post-menopausal women, osteoporosis can be reduced by weight training twice a week. Such exercise increases bone density. It also improves strength and balance, and thereby reduces the risk of falls in the elderly. This lowers the mortality rate because fractured hips from falls are associated with a fairly high death rate.

❏ A 1994 study in the *Journal of the American Medical Association* points to a decreased incidence of gastrointestinal hemorrhage among elderly people who exercise regularly.

❏ A recent article in the *Archives of Internal Medicine* demonstrated that men who were physically unfit were almost *three times as likely to die from ALL CAUSES, including cancer,* even after the researchers accounted for age, smoking, and alcohol use.

❏ Studies have shown that exercise reduces the incidence of both breast and ovarian cancer by a very significant margin, and colon cancer by 50 percent.

❏ Impotence occurs in 25 percent of all men over the age of 65. Researchers say, however, that men who regularly exercise have a much lower incidence of this problem. **If you like sex, you're going to love exercise**!

❏ Exercise is the healthiest way to treat depression. A study reported in the journal *Psychosomatic Medicine* in 2000 concluded that exercise provides as much effectiveness against depression as the latest medications. And with no side effects! Additionally, patients who exercised actually had better long term results than those on medication. After six months, medicated patients had a three times greater relapse rate than the individuals who exercised!

❏ Exercise also helps keep Alzheimer's at bay, as well as the "usual" mental decline associated with aging. It is also a very effective treatment for insomnia.

Exercise - It's Addictive

Getting sedentary patients to exercise is often a challenge. Sometimes it's harder than getting them to make any other lifestyle change.

But just try to get them to stop once they are into it for a few months.

It is truly addicting, and improves the quality of life more than any other lifestyle habit.

What Kind Of Exercise
And How Much Is Best for You?

Anti-aging specialists and researchers have been asking this question for years. Now, using the measurements derived from Bio-Energy Testing™, it is possible to precisely prescribe an individual exercise program for people of all ages, and with all conditions.

My experience gleaned from analyzing the Bio-Energy Testing™ results of hundreds of patients has taught me that aerobic (cardiovascular) exercise has a different effect on various physiological functions than does resistance (weight) training. It turns out that *both* are needed to obtain optimum results.

"Circuit training," when properly carried out, represents an exciting way to combine both aerobic and resistance training. It will save you time while simultaneously offering the best possible results.

Briefly stated, circuit training involves the use of multi-set, high repetition, non-stop weight resistance training. You adjust the resistance in order to bring your heart rate up to your optimal exercise zone, that is, between your FBR (maximum fat burning heart rate) and your ATR (anaerobic threshold heart rate). Using a heart rate monitor, if you find that your heart rate goes above your ATR, then you decrease the weight resistance. If you find that it is lower than your FBR, you increase the resistance. If you are not familiar with weight training you will definitely need a trainer to get you started, and to periodically check up on how you're doing. Most health clubs are staffed with trainers who can help you establish a circuit training program designed to keep you in your zone.

Circuit training is most effective when performed within the following parameters:

❏ Exercise the muscles of the arms, chest, back, abdomen, and, most importantly, the legs. The program should include arm curls, military presses, bench presses, pull ups, abdominal crunches, and squats or lunges.

❏ For each exercise, perform 3-4 sets of 25 repetitions each, one after another.

❏ Your heart rate zone during the entire exercise period should be in between your FBR and your ATR. The only exception is if you were briefly to go above your ATR at the end of a set. Ideally the weights should be adjusted so that time spent above your ATR is minimal.

❑ At the end of each set, wait until your heart rate has dropped to your FBR before starting the next set.

❑ Exercise for 35-40 minutes.

Are You Exercising Too Hard?

Many people, especially those who find it hard to control their weight, are actually exercising too hard for their level of fitness and genetics. Often they rely on calculated heart rate formulas that are notoriously inaccurate for individuals who are overweight. If you calculate your exercise level in this manner you are probably wasting much if not *all* of your effort.

These formulas are all based soley on age, and fail to take your genetics, body build, and level of fitness into consideration. Currently, the most widely used formulas by exercise experts to compute an individual's FBR and ATR are:

$$FBR = .65 \times [208 - (.07 \times age)]$$
$$ATR = .85 \times [208 - (.07 \times age)]$$

Let's take these formulas and apply it to one of my many real life overweight patients for whom the formulas were very misleading. Her name is Mary. Mary was forty-five years old when she first consulted a trainer to help her lose weight. Using the above formulas Mary's trainer determined her FBR to be equal to 114 beats per minute and her ATR to be 150 beats per minute.

Armed with this information, Mary's trainer instructed her to exercise at a heart rate of between 114 and 150 beats per minute.

When we measured Mary's actual zones using Bio-Energy Testing™ analysis, not surprisingly we discovered a very different picture from what had been predicted by the equations. Her FBR turned out to be 95 beats per minute, not 114, and her ATR was measured at 110 beats per minute, much lower than the predicted value of 150. **When she was working out in the zone given to her by her trainer, she was not only completely wasting her time, she was, in fact, exercising at a rate that was unhealthy and damaging for her!** Let me explain.

Burning Carbs Instead Of Fat

Mary's trainer predicted that her FBR, the rate at which she burns maximum fat, was 114 beats per minute. But Bio-Energy Testing™ determined that when she worked out at this predicted FBR, she was actually exercising above her ATR, and so was not burning any fat at all.

Remember that the ATR is where no fat is being burned, only carbohydrate stores. *When she was supposed to be burning fat, she was instead depleting her carbohydrate stores.*

Technically speaking, her drained carbohydrate stores should be replenished after exercise by her fat stores and in this way she would burn at least some fat. **But this scenario turns out to be inaccurate for one simple reason: obese persons are unable to mobilize fat stores to replenish anything!**

The only way an obese person can replenish carbohydrate stores is by eating carbohydrate. So, with depleted carbohydrates from exercise, and her blood sugar accordingly low, Mary immediately had to ingest carbohydrates in order to recover and feel well.

Thus it's not her fat stores that are replenishing her depleted carbohydrates. Instead, it's her diet. All this was reflected in Mary's statement when she first saw me: "I don't understand. No matter how hard I exercise it does no good at all. All I do is get sore, and I can't lose weight."

Pain = No Gain

The reason Mary is so sore after exercise is because her trainer had also instructed her to spend half of her exercise time at her supposed ATR of 150. But from her exercise analysis we were able to determine that her real ATR was 110, not 150. Any time she exercised above 110, which she had been doing for 25-30 minutes every day, she was going into lactic acidosis!

Lactic acidosis refers to the excessive amount of acid accumulation that occurs when people are not able to meet their energy needs by aerobic metabolism. **In individuals with optimum energy parameters it only occurs with very intense exercise, but in many people it can occur simply by walking across the room!** The tendency to go into lactic acidosis is increased by age, obesity, disease, nutrient deficiency, hormonal deficiencies, or any of the many other factors described in this book that disrupt the body's ability to produce energy.

The pain from lactic acidosis does *not* equal any gain, contrary to the popular saying. She was suffering unnecessarily. She was also increasing free radical damage to her entire body. Exercising above a heart rate of 110 not only doesn't help her lose weight or enhance her health at all, it actually will make her more susceptible to disease and injury from over-training.

Because she had been using formulas that were completely inaccurate at predicting her exercise zone, her *entire* exercise time had been wasted.

Getting Your Zone Right

As soon as Mary had completed her Bio-Energy Testing™ I was able to explain to her why she had been so unsuccessful.

"You mean I have been exercising too hard for my own good?" she asked.

"Yes," I answered. "Research is continually showing that exercise at or below the ATR is a much more effective way to lose weight and stay healthy than the old 'push-it-to-the-limits' approach."

Since she needed to lose some fat, I started her on a daily program of 45-60 minutes of walking at a pace fast enough to keep her heart rate at her true FBR of 95 beats per minute. Although the intensity of the exercise seemed minimal after all she had been through, Mary started losing about a pound of weight a week.

More importantly, she was feeling more energetic and sleeping better. Her craving for carbohydrates was gone.

In six months she lost all her excess fat. We performed another analysis at this time and found her FBR had improved to 112 beats per minute, and her ATR had risen to 130 beats per minute.

While these numbers were not yet where they needed to be for optimal anti-aging, they did demonstrate that her overall program was working. Her new FBR and ATR called for an adjusted exercise zone, which she immediately began to incorporate into her exercise program.

Within the next twelve months, her numbers became optimal, and she settled into an easy maintenance program consisting of exercise for 20-25 minutes at her ATR, three to four times per week.

Living In Lactic Acidosis

Many trainers used to using fitness formulas instead of Bio-Energy Testing™ may find the above case hard to believe. They think that it would become quickly obvious to anyone that they were in lactic acidosis since lactic acidosis causes such a characteristic rapid breathing and muscle aching. But my experience with Bio-Energy Testing™ has shown me that a large percentage of people, particularly those with weight control issues, have trained their bodies to be so used to lactic acidosis, that they don't pay much attention to these symptoms.

Because their E.Q. is so low they may spend a considerable part of their day in lactic acidosis simply from every day exertions like walking. Some of my patients go into lactic acidosis simply by getting out of a chair!! **In such people the liver often develops an extraordinary ability to convert lactic acid back to blood sugar with incredible efficiency. This allows them to spend significant amounts of their day in lactic acidosis *without* having the characteristically severe symptoms.**

Mary had been regularly exercising in lactic acidosis for over 2 years under the advice of a trainer who used the standard formulas. Exercise for her was not fun, and she had to force herself to do it. She was chronically tired and achy, but because her doctors could find no reason for these symptoms, she had just learned to live with it, and even stopped complaining about it.

Being In The Zone Is Fun

Not long after Bio-Energy Testing™ discovered her correct zones, she called me up *complaining* about her new exercise program.

"This is much too easy for me," she said. "It can't possibly work. I'm sure I'm wasting my time."

I assured her that this was because for the past two years she had been overdoing it, and naturally it felt too easy. I told her to enjoy the fact that she would no longer have to dread her exercise sessions, and that she would actually begin to look forward to them. **Exercising in the correct zone is fun and enjoyable.**

When she returned to the clinic two months later, she was smiling and finally seeing the light. She was experiencing the first non-dieting weight loss in her life.

Mary's case exemplifies the importance of exercising in your real zone, not an imaginary one deduced from one-size-fits-all formulas. I have seen so many cases like this over the years that I often wonder if these formulas actually work for anyone at all. Knowing your real FBR and ATR are invaluable keys to getting the most from your workouts. Fortunately using Bio-Energy Testing™ these values are not calculated, they are actually measured.

My 5/10 Rule

How many times have you arrived at your regularly scheduled exercise program only to find that you just don't feel up to it? I don't know about you, but this happens to me about 50 percent of the time.

My inner voice is rebelling: "I'm too tired" or "I just don't feel like it right now."

A long time ago I decided I had to develop a way of dealing with this in order to pursue any semblance of a regular exercise schedule. So I came up with what I call my 5-10 rule. It works for me. See if it works as well for you.

It goes like this:

No matter how you feel, start your exercise. *Just do it.*

If, after five minutes you actually feel worse than you did when you started, call it quits for the day

If after ten minutes, you don't feel better than you did before you started, you can also stop.

I can honestly tell you that when you use this "yardstick," you'll end up quitting only a very small percentage of the time. It just reaffirms in my mind the incredible impact of exercise on both the physical and mental level.

My Recommendations:

❑ Optimally, obtain a Bio-Energy Testing™ analysis. You can find a testing™ facility by going to www.bursting-with-energy.com on the Internet, or by calling toll free 1-866-376-0610. Determine your FBR and your ATR. Your optimum exercise zone is between these values. Unless you plan on competitive racing, there is no benefit to exercising higher than your ATR, and there may be several disadvantages. Similarly, exercising below your FBR will yield relatively little benefit.

❑ Purchase a heart rate monitor from a sporting goods store. You can buy a good device for approximately $100. Use it every time you exercise.

❑ If you don't have Bio-Energy Testing™ available, how can you tell if your exercise program is working optimally for you? A good clue is that most people start becoming breathless when they approach their ATR. The recommendation is to exercise at a rate just lower than that. Let's say you're on the treadmill. You start gradually increasing your speed. Very soon you will start huffing and puffing. At this point look at your heart rate monitor. The reading is close to your ATR. Multiply this estimated ATR by .60 to guestimate your FBR.

❑ If you need to lose weight, exercise for at least 45 to 60 minutes each day, and spend between 80 to 100 percent of your exercise effort at your FBR. If you don't need to lose weight, exercise for 25 to 30 minutes 4 or 5 times per week at your ATR.

❑ Also be sure to check your Bio-Energy Testing™ values at least once a year. As you get in better shape both your FBR and your ATR are likely to change.

Secret No. 7
Breathing For Energy

Modern science has given us all the physiological details that occur in the breathing process, but ancient thinkers had already put attention on this issue long before we had such detailed understanding. The ancients quite naturally reasoned that since_not breathing was synonymous with death, breathing itself must be pretty important, and furthermore, there must be both proper and improper ways to breathe.

It turns out that they were quite right.

There is a right way to breathe and a wrong way. And all too frequently we do it wrong. **Improper breathing is, in fact, a major - and widely ignored - cause of stress, panic attacks, anxiety, low energy, and premature aging.** This became very clear to me soon after I began using Bio-Energy Testing™ analysis in my clinic.

A primary example was Steve, a 43-year-old patient who made his living installing dry wall. In order to be successful in a very competitive field he worked hard, long hours. He first consulted me about low energy and episodes that his previous doctors called panic attacks. When they occurred, he felt as though he could not catch a complete breath. His heart would beat rapidly. He would become fearful of passing out.

These episodes occurred suddenly and without warning. He had stopped drinking his usual daily pot of coffee, but the problem nevertheless persisted. Other doctors told him that testing revealed no abnormality, and that the drop in his energy level was probably just secondary to a "generalized anxiety disorder."

Steve was prescribed an anti-depressant medication, and told to work at a less stressful occupation. He came to our clinic looking for another answer.

Bio-Energy Testing™ testing revealed a fairly significant decrease in energy production secondary to insufficient oxygen delivery at the capillary level. This clearly explained the low energy and decreased stamina. At rest his respiration rate was between fifteen to eighteen breaths per minute.

Most importantly, Steve breathed by expanding his chest, even when lying down. This is fairly unusual because while lying down most people automatically breathe with the abdomen in what is known as *diaphragmatic or abdominal breathing.*

Steve hadn't noticed any shortness of breath. He said his breathing seemed normal.

Immediately after the testing, my technician spent a half-hour teaching Steve proper breathing techniques. Then we re-examined his Bio-Energy Testing™. We found that the respiration rate came down to under twelve per minute, and his energy production *increased 20 percent to an almost optimum level.*

The turnaround occurred in less than one hour, simply the result of breathing properly.

The most significant development was the rapid relief of his so-called "generalized anxiety disorder." After just three weeks of practicing breathing exercises for fifteen minutes twice a day, Steve's anxiety symptoms virtually disappeared. And along with this, he experienced a major increase in energy.

Such dramatic results, and in such a short period of time, demonstrates how powerful an influence breathing habits can have on our quality of life. Steve's case is not really all that unusual. After years of seeing patients diagnosed with chronic anxiety and panic disorder, I am firmly convinced that many of these problems result simply from improper breathing.

The Right and Wrong Way to Breathe

There are two, really quite different ways to breathe:

❑ Chest wall breathing

Chest wall breathing employs the chest, shoulder, and neck muscles to lift up the chest in order to inflate the lungs. As you inhale, the chest expands. The abdomen is sucked in.

This is the classic "chest out, abdomen in" form of breathing taught in the military and reinforced in our culture all throughout youth. To determine if you are a "chest breather," just sit quietly in a chair, resting and breathing easily, and observe how your chest and abdomen move when you inhale. If your abdomen does not go out every time you inhale, and/or if your chest expands, you are chest breathing. This is not the preferred "style."

Steve was a habitual chest wall breather. As we will discuss in a moment, there are several reasons why this type of breathing aggravates and even causes chronic anxiety.

❑ Diaphragmatic or "abdominal" breathing

If your abdomen bulges out when you inhale and your chest remains still, that's diaphragmatic breathing. It means you are using the diaphragm, an internal muscle located at the bottom of the chest cage, to draw in the air. As the diaphragm expands downward, the abdomen naturally expands along with it. This is the preferred "style."

The Shortcomings of Chest Wall Breathing

Chest wall breathing fails to draw in as much oxygen into the lung's air sacks as does abdominal breathing.

Here's why: The lungs have what is known in pulmonary physiology as "dead space." This refers simply to the space taken up by the tubes (airways) through which the air passes en route to the air sacks, where oxygen is delivered to the bloodstream. The airways are thus "dead space" in that they don't participate in the actual oxygen exchange. It turns out that the upper part of the lungs has more dead space than the lower part.

Chest wall breathing selectively fills the upper part of the lungs. Abdominal breathing selectively fills the lower part. Thus, the former is less efficient in the mechanics of oxygen acquisition.

In order to make up for the decreased amount of oxygen acquired per breath, chest wall breathers automatically compensate by increasing their respiratory rate. At rest, Steve's rate was typical of this: twelve to eighteen breaths per minute. By comparison, an abdominal breather usually needs only six to eight breaths per minute to acquire the same volume of oxygen.

Chest wall breathers are obviously working harder to acquire the same amount of oxygen as an abdominal breather. That's only part of the downside.

The increased respiratory rate associated with chest wall breathing is known as "chronic sub-acute hyperventilation." It can be clearly detected by Bio-Energy Testing™ analysis because it results in an excessive excretion of carbon dioxide. The increased loss of carbon dioxide shifts the pH of the blood in the brain and in the rest of the body into a state known as **alkalosis**, often leading to chronic, unexplained anxiety.

Alkalosis also results in a decreased oxygen delivery to every cell in your body. Let me explain how.

As I explained in Chapter 2, when you breath in oxygen it gets taken up by the hemoglobin molecule contained in your red blood cells. Hemoglobin has an incredibly strong attraction for oxygen. It holds tightly to the oxygen as it passes though the arterial network and down to the level of the cells, where oxygen is delivered.

The hemoglobin molecule is triggered to release its oxygen cargo in response to the acid pH it encounters at the cellular level. However, the normal acid pH becomes disrupted due to the alkalosis caused by chest wall breathing. This state of affairs effectively prevents the hemoglobin molecule from releasing its oxygen. The result is a decrease in available oxygen to the cells, and a decrease in energy production.

This is why Steve, and others like him, suffer from low energy.

If you have ever gone through a very stressful period - and who hasn't - you may have noticed that afterward you feel drained and fatigued. One reason for this is that stress almost always puts people into a chest wall breathing mode. And, as you've just read, this contributes to low energy through the alkalosis effect.

Since the physiology is designed to operate more efficiently through abdominal breathing, you might be wondering why our bodies developed the ability to chest wall breathe. The answer has to do with how and when the brain senses peril.

Under emergency situations, at times of danger, the body requires additional oxygen. In the distant past you would have needed a major injection of oxygen to flee from a lion that had targeted you for its next meal. To meet such threatening challenges, the body kicks into a double breathing mode: chest wall combined with abdominal breathing. This quickly sucks in an extra supply of oxygen.

In intense situations like these, where exertion is at an ultra peak level, alkalosis does not occur. Oxygen uptake and delivery are maximized. Thus, the body evolved the capability of chest breathing as a survival mechanism.

Although survival and escape from life-threatening predicaments may not be part of daily existence for most of us, the everyday variety of mental anguish and stresses experienced in modern living is enough to switch on the chest wall breathing response. The unconscious part of the brain reads this initiation of chest wall breathing as a sign of an impending danger, and triggers anxiety attacks.

You may just be sitting in your car worrying about running late for an appointment. Unbeknownst to you, the tension causes you to begin to chest wall breathe, and then whamo, your brain senses danger and suddenly goes into an emergency mode. You may then experience a panicky feeling, which is all the more stressful because there is no apparent reason why you should have such a reaction.

The Nitty-Gritty on Sighing

Before I close the case on chest wall breathing, I'd like to share a few comments on sighing. Although you may associate sighing with the sight of a heart-throb or other romantic imagery, the body has other primary reasons in mind. A sigh is a *distinct physiological event* characterized by a deep full breath, using both abdominal and chest wall breathing. Sighs naturally occur about every 10-15 minutes, allowing the lungs to completely fill up. At times other than when we are exerting, we use very little of our lung capacity. The body creates the sigh response - a quick, deep breath - to help expand and engage areas of the lungs not being used.

I'm sure you have had many occasions to notice the wonderfully relaxing effect of a sigh. It often seems to automatically occur when you are stressed.

One problem with chronic chest wall breathing is that due to its associated hyperventilation and alkalosis, the body is often unable to sigh. When this happens it can be very disturbing. Sometimes a patient who desires the calming benefit of a sigh, but can't pull it off as a result of chronic chest wall breathing, will call me quite concerned and say, "I can't get a deep enough breath, and I think something must be wrong with my lungs."

And, of course, the mere thought that "something is wrong with my lungs" is enough to agitate most people and maybe even trigger an anxiety attack. In these cases, I just explain some basic facts on sighing and tell the concerned patient to relax and not worry about it. First, you can only sigh a maximum of one time every ten minutes. Two, you can't force a sigh. You just have to be patient and wait for it to happen. Three, not being able to initiate a sigh at will does not indicate that there is any problem with the lungs.

Don't be nervous if you can't sigh on demand. Just be patient and wait. It will come soon enough, but only to the degree that you are breathing with your abdomen.

Breaking the Vicious Cycle

Chronic chest wall breathing generates a vicious cycle. It causes:

❑ Increased respiration

❑ Alkalosis, resulting in decreased oxygen consumption

❑ Decreased energy production

❑ Interference with the sighing mechanism

❑ An emergency mode in the body

❑ Anxiety and stress

All of this promotes even more chest breathing. And if you throw in a stressful event you can readily see how an anxiety attack can develop.

When anxiety becomes chronic, most people will run to the doctor and get a prescription for a sedative. The medication slows down the respiratory rate and seems to correct the problem. However, the sedative only takes care of the symptoms, and does not correct the root problem. Often, it creates new problems in terms of side effects.

A healthier way is to teach yourself to breathe with your diaphragm. If you're interested, and I hope you will be, the information below tells you how.

The alternative is to continue the habit of chest wall breathing, which will deprive you of optimal energy and age you faster.

How to Breathe the Right Way

Diaphragmatic breathing is one of the very first techniques that singers and musicians are taught in order to provide them with ample oxygen for those long notes. I personally learned the method years ago in a yoga class, and it gave me a significant advantage later when I was actively involved in competitive cycling.

The technique is quite simple, but you may need some guidance because it is somewhat subtle. Once you've got the idea, it just takes a little practice over a few months to fully perfect it and make it automatic.

In the beginning I made up little signs saying "breathe!" I put them everywhere. On my watch, my dashboard, my bike, my mirror. The signs were reminders to check how I was breathing.

And when I checked I was usually breathing with my chest. In that case I would just take a few good abdominal breaths, and try to concentrate on breathing this way as much as possible. The other thing I did which helped enormously was to spend a few minutes every morning and evening performing breath meditation (which I will explain in a moment).

But first follow these few simple points to learn the diaphragmatic technique. Most people can grasp the basic movement within a few minutes. Here's what to do:

❑ Lay down on your back. It's hard to chest wall breath while lying down. Even the most "die hard" chest breathers tend to breathe with the diaphragm in this position.

❑ Now place your hand on your abdomen and notice how it rises slightly when you inhale, and goes down when you exhale. *This movement is the hallmark of breathing with your diaphragm.* If you breath with your chest, your hand will not elevate during the inhale, but will instead drop down. If you are naturally breathing with your diaphragm while lying down you are well on your way. If it isn't coming naturally, don't worry. Just give it a bit more time. You'll get it soon enough.

❑ After you finally become familiar with the feel of diaphragmatic breathing, I would like you to practice an exaggerated form of it by contracting your abdominal muscles inward (sucking in your gut) as you exhale the air from your lungs.

❑ Then expand the same muscles outward to inhale.

❑ Keep practicing this technique until you can breathe fully and somewhat deeply without moving your chest.

❑ If the movement doesn't come easy, enroll the help of a spouse or friend or yoga instructor to help you.

❑ Once you learned to do this lying down, try the same thing while sitting in a chair, and then while standing. Finally, to perfect your newly discovered "talent," try doing it while you are singing in the shower or lightly exercising. You can then proudly announce to friends and family that you have finally learned to breathe correctly!

There are additional benefits to diaphragmatic breathing that should help inspire you. One is that it often helps to eliminate or significantly reduce neck pain and tension commonly caused by chronically raising up the chest during chest wall breathing. Diaphragmatic breathing does not create any neck and shoulder strain since it moves with gravity instead of against it. It also strengthens and tightens the abdominal muscles. And finally, it often benefits individuals with asthma or other lung conditions.

Breath Meditation

Perhaps nothing is as powerful as the mind to either make us sick or keep us healthy. But how can we learn to harness and direct that power? One tried and true method is breath meditation.

This meditative exercise is particularly effective against stress-related disorders, insomnia, and hypertension. It will also generate more energy and stamina. In addition, it's a very effective way *to train your mind to work better for you.* That means increased mental clarity, speed, and memory.

Moreover, breath meditation is completely free and devoid of side effects. No gyms to join or pills to take!

The little time it takes to do it will very typically lead to many wonderful rewards.

First, let's get the concept straight. Meditation, at least the way I'm using the word, refers to mental exercise. Meditation and prayer are not the same thing. Praying is a different concept. It has its own powers, but does *not* substitute for meditation. So even if you regularly pray, please be sure to practice some form of meditation as well.

Breath meditation trains the conscious mind to focus better and the unconscious mind to relax better. It works in the same way that training your muscles makes them function better.

Most of the time your meditation session will be relaxing. But there can also be days in which emotions or stresses may preoccupy your mind, and you may find yourself expending more effort to meditate. Don't worry about that. It's normal. You just take it as it comes and apply the simple guidelines I'm giving you.

What's important to understand here is that no matter how relaxing a meditation session may or may not be, it will still serve to improve your overall relaxation potential and strengthen your powers of concentration.

Your Mind Is Like A Puppy

Your mind wants to wander around and experience everything it can. This is a wonderful thing, but it can also limit the mind's ability to focus, and mental power is directly related to focus.

Breath meditation trains your mind to better focus, and in so doing strengthens your mental power. This increases the ease at which you do everything!

The process takes fifteen to twenty minutes and if you can do it regularly once or twice a day it may be the most productive fifteen or twenty minutes of "doing nothing" that you can possibly imagine.

Just follow the easy steps and you'll be on your way.

❑ **Step 1   The Setting**

First of all, you ideally need some quiet space, a room where you can meditate without interruption. If there's a phone in the room, pull out the plug.

120

You need a comfortable chair, one with arm rests if possible.

Sit comfortably. Don't cross your legs.

Take three deep relaxing breaths, and when you exhale the third time, let your eyes close.

❑ **Step 2 Breathing in Squares**

Use the diaphragmatic breathing technique you just learned.

I want you to "breathe in squares." By that I mean pausing to hold your breath both at the end of your inhale and your exhale. The pauses should be the same length of time that you use to breathe. For example, if you inhale (expanding your abdomen in the process) over a two- second period, then hold your breath for a two-second pause before you begin to exhale. Then exhale (sucking in your abdomen) over a two-second interval. At the end of your exhale pause for two seconds before you begin the next breath. If you inhale over a three-second count, then just make sure that the other intervals are three-second long.

Keep repeating this process for each and every breath. It's as simple as that!

You can count the seconds to yourself as you go along but after a while you will probably find that your are able to naturally keep the intervals the same without counting.

Just remember to breathe only with your abdomen. Keep your chest free of movement.

While you go through this routine there are two things to be aware of:

✳ Sighs and Yawns

Most people experience the need to sigh about every ten minutes as I mentioned before. During meditation, when you feel the urge to sigh, just go with it. Remember that sighing invokes both chest wall and diaphragmatic breathing.   After the sigh simply return to the abdominal breathing in squares.   Sometimes you may feel the urge to sigh but it just doesn't develop. This just means that your body doesn't need one yet. Sighs are relaxing, but don't force them. Be patient. One will come along soon enough.

Don't be bothered by yawning.   I can remember many times when I have yawned as much as twenty times in a meditation session. Just go with it, and as soon as the yawn passes simply return to abdominal breathing in squares.

✳ Altering Your Breathing Rate

One thing sure to happen while you are practicing breath meditation is that you will need to alter the breathing rate to accommodate how your feel. If you feel breathless or have "air hunger," you will need to increase the rate. This is often noticed during the pause at the end of exhalation.

When you notice this, simply increase your breathing rate so that you are comfortable and no longer feel in need of air. For example, if you are breathing in two second intervals and you feel breathless, decrease the intervals to one second. This adjustment will cause your breathing rate to increase and get rid of the breathless feeling.

Conversely, as the session progresses and your body becomes more relaxed you will usually need to *decrease* your breathing rate. If you start to feel a little dizzy as if you are hyperventilating or breathing too fast, just decrease your breathing rate accordingly by *increasing* the length of the intervals. You may very likely have to adjust your breathing rate a number of times during a session in order to keep feeling comfortable.

❑ Step 3 Training the Puppy

A crucial part of breath meditation is your mental focus. While you are just sitting there comfortably using your abdominal muscles to breathe in squares, it is important that you keep your mind entirely focused on your breathing. You can focus on your breathing rate, how the air feels in your lungs, or how your abdomen feels as it moves in and out. It doesn't make a difference exactly what you focus on, as long as it has something to do with your breathing.

But remember what I said a moment ago about the mind being like a very inquisitive and active puppy. It may not always reconcile itself with the drill called meditation.

Imagine having a puppy on a leash and training it to sit comfortably by your side. As soon as you place the puppy on the floor next to you, it will immediately begin to wander in one direction or another. Without becoming upset with the puppy, just imagine yourself gently retrieving it, and putting it next to you again.

Your mind is going to stray the same way. No matter how hard you try to keep your attention on your breathing, the mind will wander off into this thought or that thought.

Just like with the puppy, as soon as you become aware that your mind is wandering, gently retrieve it and refocus on your breathing.

This repetitive cycle of concentrating, straying, and refocusing again is the nature of breath meditation. The more you practice this retrieving and refocusing, the stronger your power of concentration will be. After several months of regular practice, you will begin to notice that the mind is wandering less, and that you are retrieving your awareness more easily. Although your mind is an extremely stubborn puppy, it will eventually learn.

People who continue meditating in this fashion see an improvement in virtually every health function measured. The practice contributes to longer and healthier life. Don't underestimate the power of this simple exercise to increase your energy levels, enhance your mental speed and concentration, and improve your mood, sleep, and emotional state.

My Recommendations:

❑ During the day, and especially when you exercise, check your breathing regularly to see if you are breathing correctly. Be patient, and keep working at it. It took me about two years before I was consistently breathing correctly without thinking about it.

❑ Make it part of your routine to practice breath meditation 15 minutes once or twice a day as your schedule allows. The best time for most people is before and after work. At first it may seem a little intimidating, but after a few months, you will actually prefer it over anything else you might have done before to unwind and relax.

Secret No. 8
Natural Hormones For Energy

U ndoubtedly the single most important contribution to the new explosion of anti-aging medicine has been the availability of natural or "bio-identical" hormones and the growing research regarding their effects.

The efficacy of *all* of the secrets I discuss in this book is often limited in the absence of proper hormonal replacement.

Hormones are molecular messengers that control healing, tissue regeneration, immune function, sexual function, memory and mood, strength, body composition, skin thickness, energy, digestion, and virtually every other aspect of human function. Most people, when they hear the word "hormone," think only of sex hormones, but there are many other hormones beside these.

Ever wonder how it is that young people can smoke, eat terrible diets, fail to get enough rest, experience huge amounts of stress, and still do better than older folks who are taking much beter care of themselves? Well, wonder no more. It's about hormones. Youth is a time of boundless levels of hormones. And as we navigate through the years, the hormone tank becomes drained.

Refilling the tank has become an exciting new frontier in medicine, which I am thrilled to be part of. And refilling the tank, that is, replacing drained hormones, often produces such startling reversals in energy production and overall health that patients can't believe all the good things that are happening to them.

I am not just limiting this conversation to restoring deficient levels of estrogen or progesterone for menopausal women. For sure, this has significant benefits. I am talking of replacing many different hormones in both women and men as they get older.

Here are some of the common improvements I see as a result of this approach:

❑ Significant increase in energy

❑ Increased exercise capacity

❑ Enhanced sexual performance

❑ Strengthening of the heart, liver, spleen, kidneys, brain, and other organs that atrophy with aging

❑ Improved cardiac function

❑ Fat loss *without dieting*

❑ Increased muscle mass *without exercising*

❑ Blood pressure regulation

❑ Reduction of wrinkles and tighter, thicker skin

❑ Better mood and sleep

❑ Increased mental function

❑ Enhanced healing

❑ Stronger bones

❑ Lower LDL cholesterol, the so-called "bad cholesterol," that contributes to harmful plaque when it becomes oxidized

❑ Better resistance against infections and illness

Hormonal Replacement Is The Key

Just over a decade ago, Daniel Rudman, M.D, of the Medical College of Wisconsin, published a landmark study in the New England Journal of Medicine showing that six months of human growth hormone replacement significantly reduced body fat, increased muscle mass, and improved every cardiac and pulmonary function measured.

A decreased muscle to fat ratio is a hallmark of aging. So what Rudman concluded is that he essentially **reversed the functional age of his patients ten to twenty years simply by restoring their growth hormone levels to youthful levels!**

As hard to believe as that result is, Rudman based his conclusion on results obtained from sound scientific principles verified by a highly controlled medical study.

Growth hormone, of course, is only *one* of the hormones that become deficient as we age. How much better might his results might have been if he had simultaneously replaced other deficient hormones, and placed his patients on an optimum diet, supplement, and lifestyle program, including attention to exercise, sunlight, water, and sleep.

> **The major difference between you at age fifty and you at age twenty-five is hormonal**.

After the end of our reproductive age, generally around thirty-five (but in some cases even earlier), the body's production of hormones starts a steady decline. It's a dirty trick that Nature plays on us. It's as if to say, well, you have reproduced to ensure the perpetuation of the species, so you're not really needed any more.

The question is not if we are going to become hormone deficient, it is rather a question of when, and how significant the deficiencies will be. The rate at which these deficiencies develop determines how fast we will age, and the major determining factors are genetics and lifestyle. More than any other single factor, the hormonal deficiencies that routinely occur as we get older are the cause of the deterioration, diseases, and symptoms of aging.

Hormones Are Not Just A Female Thing

Hormonal deficiencies affect both men and women. We are specifically aware of twelve different hormones in women and eight in men that become deficient as we age. The symptoms they create include hair loss, fatigue, weakness, decreased stamina, decreased muscle mass, decreased sexual drive and function, insomnia, depression, anxiety, reduced mental function, wrinkles, increased fat mass, bladder disorders, decreased bone mass, declining immune system function, reduced equilibrium, and above all, decreased energy production.

Hormone deficiency symptoms such as constipation, headaches, infertility, and menstrual disturbances can occur even in younger people. Although symptoms of deficiencies usually don't show up until we're in our forties or fifties, it is not uncommon for me to see the signs in patients as young as twenty. Occasionally, I even see them in children.

Hormonal deficiencies play a major role in the development of virtually every age related disease including cancer, stroke, heart disease, osteoporosis, arthritis, depression, Alzheimer's dementia, and diabetes.

Now that's the bad news.

The good news is that recent advances in scientific technology allow us to accurately test for hormonal deficiencies and replace them with natural or bio-identical hormones. By the term natural and bio-identical, I mean manmade hormones that are exact molecular replicas of your own hormones.

With these two advances, hormone replacement has joined the 21st century.

There are many long-term and short- term studies with both men and women which demonstrate the effectiveness of hormone replacement. **Subjects live longer and have a much greater quality of life than those not supplemented**. Using natural hormone replacement we can safely and naturally treat hormonal deficiencies as they develop.

It's Never Too Late

Jane had many health problems when she first came to me as a new patient. Although she was only 74-years-old, she had severe chronic lung disease from years of smoking, and could barely walk across the room without help. Her heart was also starting to fail and her bones had become quite osteoporotic. Besides her chronic shortness of breath, her main complaint was profound weakness. She took several medications to help her breathe better and was dependent on a supply of oxygen at all times.

Jane, like many other older people, had been told by her medical doctor to "learn to live with it" because "at your age you should be content just to be alive." Unfortunately, a great many physicians and patients subscribe to the concept that being weak and feeble are just inevitable features of being older.

I told Jane when I first saw her that her lung disease was permanent, and that it could not be repaired. However, I added, it was very possible to improve her energy production and hence her overall health by giving her body back the hormones it had been missing for thirty years or more.

Within three months we had Jane following a comprehensive natural hormonal replacement program that included estrogens, progesterone, testosterone, melatonin, thyroid, DHEA, and growth hormone. She was also taught how to breathe properly, placed on a high protein diet with a broad range program of nutritional supplements, and given an individualized exercise program.

In a few short months, she showed considerable improvement in energy, pain, strength, and sleep. She still needed to carry her oxygen bottle around with her wherever she went, but she was now able to readily go up the same flight of stairs in her home that had previously been extremely difficult for her.

Now, three years later, instead of being worse off, Jane has made significant improvements across-the-board. Her lung condition has not degenerated. Her bone density is better. Her heart function is better. Had it not been for hormonal replacement, it is quite possible that she would either have been dead or institutionalized. I'll leave it to you to figure out which is worse.

Such improvements, even in someone with poor health, are not unusual. One of the characteristics of natural hormone replacement is that the so-called "natural" deterioration associated with aging seems to go into reverse gear.

How Are Hormonal Deficiencies Determined?

As in Jane's case, and with other patients, hormonal deficiencies are determined in three different ways. First, a detailed history and physical examination can often lead to suspicion of a specific deficiency.

Afterward, laboratory testing confirms or negates the connection.

Finally, a therapeutic trial can be initiated to see if specific symptoms resolve with proper replacement.

A word about laboratory testing for hormonal disorders. Properly monitoring hormone levels is almost a specialty in itself. Newer, more sensitive laboratory methods are being continually developed that are better able to identify deficiencies in a patient who may have tested within normal range using less precise assessments. For this reason, I use several laboratories, some of them even located outside of the United States, to give me the best possible chance to assess patients.

Blood tests are notoriously limited in assessing hormonal problems. That's due to the rapid fluctuations of hormone levels in the blood, and also because blood levels often don't accurately reflect the levels of hormones out in the tissues, where they are working.

Currently, the best method for assessing most hormone levels is by testing saliva. Saliva testing is easier on the patient and also much less expensive. It's not perfect by any means. No test is. But it seems to be more helpful than blood testing. For thyroid assessment, the most sensitive method is Bio-Energy Testing™.

What's So Different About "Natural" Hormone Replacement?

Natural hormone replacement refers to the use of hormones which are molecularly identical to those that already exist in the body. Unfortunately these "bio-identical" hormones have not been commercially available until recently, and many physicians still prescribe synthetic hormones. Synthetic hormonal therapy is still the conventional way hormones are replaced, but it has some serious drawbacks.

Drawback No 1: Synthetic hormones are not really hormones at all. In reality, they are drugs with hormone-like effects. These commonly prescribed substances are *not* found in the human body. They are *molecularly different* from the hormones they are replacing.

Since they are foreign to the body, they not only cannot function properly, but are also treated by the liver as toxins. According to several studies on the use of these synthetic hormones, side effects prompt up to 30 percent of all patients to stop using them within twelve months.

All this begs the question: "If I am deficient in a particular hormone, why isn't the deficiency treated with that exact hormone?"

Unfortunately, the reason has nothing to do with good medicine, or even common sense. The answer lies in the fact that molecules that occur naturally in the body such as hormones, are not patentable, and hence not as profitable to sell as patented drugs.

The good news, however, is that natural hormone therapy - using replacements that are molecularly identical to the hormones in the body - can be prescribed for patients through many doctors aware of their use. Although they cost a little more, they are very definitely worth it.

Drawback No 2: The conventional approach often ignores the fact that hormones work together as a team. Although each individual hormone has it's own specific actions, it also requires other hormones to be present in order to properly function. **Since any given hormone can enhance the action of one hormone while suppressing another, too much or too little of one hormone can create an imbalance in other hormones.**

The system of hormonal checks and balances is the way the body regulates itself. If a person is deficient in two hormones, he or she should replace both hormones. If seven hormones are deficient, all seven should be replaced for optimum results. Conventional replacement strategy fails to recognize these relationships.

Drawback No 3: The conventional approach tends to embrace a "one size fits all" mentality. Individual hormone deficiencies vary greatly. Therefore, the correct dose for one patient with a particular hormone deficiency may be very different from another patient.

It is quite common for patients to take either too much or too little hormone in the conventional approach.

The only reliable way to discover these differences is to monitor each patient's response with a series of hormone tests and clinical evaluations, both before and during replacement therapy.

My Three Golden Rules

To avoid these problems, I follow "three golden rules" in regard to hormone replacement and they have worked well for me over the years.

Golden Rule No. 1: I use only natural (molecularly identical) hormones that are normally found in the human body. For example, it has never made any sense to me to replace the human hormone estradiol, an estrogen compound, with the horse hormones that comprise Premarin®, the common estrogen prescription for women.

Similarly, since natural progesterone is available, and is identical to the body's own progesterone, why use a substitute drug like medroxyprogesterone acetate, commonly sold as Provera®? But this is what many physicians still use.

Foreign substances such as Provera® set off immune responses in the body that frequently cause complications.

The complications so commonly seen with synthetic hormones simply don't occur when natural hormones are used.

Golden Rule No. 2: Using comprehensive laboratory hormonal assessment, I replace *each and every* hormonal deficiency present. This helps maintain a more youthful balance of hormones.

Golden Rule No. 3: I individualize all doses. I prescribe just enough, and not too much of each hormone being replaced in each individual case. One size definitely does not fit all. Even twins may have widely divergent levels of hormones that are normal for each. A particular hormone level that is high for one person could be too low for another. This phenomenon is referred to as biochemical individuality.

Sensitive laboratory testing helps accommodate the need to respect individuality. The process is greatly helped along by feedback from patients.

Everybody is different, so it's unreasonable to expect that the same dose of a hormone will be appropriate in all cases. Because of this fact, almost all hormone replacement capsules and creams are made up individually for each patient.

The process of making a customized capsule or cream for a particular patient is called "compounding." Such customized medications are available only from what are known as "compounding pharmacies." These pharmacies specialize in making hormone prescriptions, and other preparations, directly from raw materials and according to the exact recommendations of a physician.

At pharmacies which are not compounding pharmacies, you are only able to obtain the standard one-size-fits-all dosages supplied by drug manufacturers.

Is It Safe *Not* To Replace Hormonal Deficiencies?

The most frequent question I hear from patients regarding natural replacement of deficient hormones is the obvious one: Is it safe?

I believe it is among the safest of all medical treatments. Moreover, I tell my patients that the most significant danger regarding hormonal replacement is *not* replacing your depleted hormones.

And so I pose the following question: Is it safe *not* to replace hormonal deficiencies?

Although the scientific and clinical data on this issue can be criticized from all sides, in my mind the evidence is incontrovertible: denying a patient natural hormonal replacement is dangerous.

For example, in *every* long-term human study published which looked at estrogen replacement therapy, the patients on estrogen replacement lived longer, had a lower incidence of disease, and had a higher quality of life than comparison groups who did not take the hormone.

According to one published study of 8881 post-menopausal women, *"current users with more than 15 years of estrogen use had a 40 percent reduction in their overall mortality."* The users also had a reduced mortality from cancer.

In another study that evaluated elderly men on testosterone replacement therapy, the researchers found no side effects related to the prostate. What's more, they found that the treatment had a positive impact on cholesterol that they felt reduced the risk of death from cardiovascular disease.

These gratifying results occurred in spite of the fact that the research was done with synthetic hormone drugs. One can only wonder how much better the results would have been had the hormones been natural.

Several short-term human studies have demonstrated that replacement with natural hormones generates a host of significant rejuvenating effects, particularly improved energy and an increased sense of well being. Animal studies have repeatedly demonstrated that animals whose depleted hormones are normalized lived substantially longer, and had much greater energy and vitality.

About Estrogens

Estrogen is not one, but actually three hormone compounds that have played a dominant role in the medical research and application of hormone replacement therapy. For that reason I'll be referring in the text to the plural "estrogens".

In most people's minds, the word "hormone" is synonymous with estrogens.

The reason is quite simple. The estrogens are the most powerful hormones in the female body. Virtually every cell membrane has receptor sites (areas of activity) specific for estrogens.

These compounds affect everything from the way a woman thinks to the way she looks. They exert a profound influence on the bladder, brain, soft tissues of the joints and muscles, arteries, liver, bones, fat cells, the thyroid gland, and cellular metabolism in general.

Estrogens cause a marked improvement in the HDL/LDL cholesterol ratio, keep the blood thin, and decrease the clotting tendency of the blood. They are the reason that heart attacks and strokes occur much less frequently in women.

They are also extremely powerful antioxidants, and in this way retard the aging process in general.

They stimulate the synthesis of choline acetyl-transferase, an important brain enzyme that is lacking in Alzheimer's disease. Thus, a deficiency of estrogens is regarded as a primary cause of this disease in women. Even without the extreme of outright Alzheimer's disease, a deficiency of the estrogens results in mood swings, forgetfulness, and difficulty in concentration.

The wrinkles that begin to develop after menopause are primarily secondary to a deficiency in estrogens because the hormones enhance the production of collagen and keep the skin thick and hydrated. Estrogens also prevent the facial hair growth that is common after menopause.

As you will see in the last chapter, a deficiency of estrogen not only causes osteoporosis, but is also behind many of the other diseases associated with aging women.

Lastly, and perhaps more importantly, according to Uzzi Reiss, M.D., author of a fabulous book entitled *"Natural Hormone Balance For Women,"* females with estrogen deficiency frequently speak of a decreased sense of "woman-ness." They often report a lower self-image, sexuality, and sensuality.

Half The Death Rate

One of the most famous studies on the benefits of estrogens came out of the Oakland (California) Kaiser Permanente Medical Care Program in 1996. The study monitored 232 women who for years had been taking estradiol, the most potent estrogen compound. These women were compared with a "control group" of other women who did not take any hormones.

The results showed that women taking the estradiol had nearly *half* the overall death rate of those who didn't! Deaths from cancer were essentially the same in both groups.

Despite this study and others like it, estrogen replacement therapy (ERT) has received a rash of criticism that it doesn't quite deserve. The criticism stems mostly from the fact that ERT, *as it is conventionally administered,* produces a slightly increased risk for breast cancer. ERT decreases the risk of other cancers, but because the incidence of breast cancer is so high these days, even a tiny increase in the risk is worrisome.

In my practice I routinely recommend ERT to my women patients. But not ERT as is conventionally administered.

Conventional ERT uses synthetic hormones. I use only natural hormones in my practice. There is *no* evidence they have the same effect.

The difference between these two approaches - natural and conventional - is very significant. For starters, conventional replacement therapy isn't replacement therapy at all. It's drug therapy.

The definition of the term "replacement therapy" infers that a deficient molecule is replaced by an identical molecule. But conventional ERT often involves Premarin® or other patented drug substitutes, which are bio-chemically different from the hormones they are supposed to be replacing. Premarin®, for example, contains horse estrogens. It has no human estrogens at all.

As my good friend Jonathan Wright, M.D., a pioneer in the science of natural hormonal replacement has been saying for years, "Premarin® is replacement therapy for horses, but it is drug therapy for humans."

No wonder Premarin® and the other synthetic estrogens can cause problems in humans. They don't belong in the human body. **So far there has been absolutely no study indicating that replacement of estrogens with identical human estrogens has a negative effect on breasts or any other part of the female body**.

A reasonable person may ask, "If human estrogens are available, why are physicians prescribing Premarin® and other synthetic estrogens?"

Once again, the answer has absolutely nothing to do with good medicine. Not even the most brilliant physician could justify the practice. The reason is not medical. It is economic. It stems from the fact that the law does not allow pharmaceutical companies to patent a substance that is naturally occurring. The pharmaceutical industry is a multi-billion dollar, for-profit corporate industry, and like any other industry its primary interest is the bottom line.

And since the FDA demands very extensive tests and clinical investigations before any pharmaceutical treatment can be approved, it does not make good business sense to market a non-patentable substance. The end result of this "catch 22" situation is that you receive a patentable combination containing horse estrogens or other synthetics instead of the real thing.

A Balancing Act

Another problem with conventional prescriptions of estrogens relates to lack of balance. There are three estrogen compounds in the body, as I mentioned before. They go by the names estradiol, estrone, and estriol. Estradiol is the most powerful, and in the body, estrone and estriol interact with estradiol and keep it in check. This is the body's intelligence at work. It's a balancing act. Balance is critical to hormones, because they have such major effects in the body. So there is a reason that Nature put three estrogens in the body, and not just one.

To replace an estradiol deficiency with estradiol, but neglect to replace an estriol or estrone deficiency doesn't make good sense. Moreover, it can be quite dangerous.

The pharmaceutical companies have patented a delivery system called the estradiol patch to enhance the introduction of the compound into the body. There has been much advertising hoopla about this new form of ERT because the product actually uses the natural form of estradiol. However, the problem with the estradiol patch is that it is not balanced with estrone and estriol.

When I prescribe ERT to my patients, I prescribe all three compounds in a balanced formula. They are natural, and bio-identical to what a woman has in her body. And I always individualize the dose for each woman based on testing and retesting of her hormonal status in order to maintain that balance.

Creams vs. Pills

Another important consideration regarding natural ERT is how the estrogens are being administered. It turns out that estrogens taken in the form of pills or capsules upset the balance of other hormones such as growth hormone and thyroid hormones. Oral estrogen has this effect because it tends to bind up the hormone-carrying protein known as "sex hormone binding globulin."

This "carrier" protein is formed in the liver. It not only carries estrogens around the body, but it also carries the thyroid hormones and growth hormone. When oral estrogens are used, they tend to use up the globulin to the point that it can't carry as much of these other hormones. The net effect is that the production of these hormones becomes reduced.

For this reason, whenever possible, I prefer to use topical creams over estrogen capsules and pills. The creams bind up much less sex hormone binding globulin because they pass through the skin rather than the liver.

About Progesterone

Progesterone is a critical hormone in the reproductive cycle. After a woman ovulates, she produces progesterone in the ovaries to prepare the uterus for conception and the development of the fertilized egg.

But progesterone also plays many other key protective roles in a woman's body. It accomplishes the following:

- ❑ Helps to balance the estrogen compounds.

- ❑ Provides hormonal security against the formation of breast and uterine cancer.

- ❑ Acts as a natural diuretic, and as such decreases edema and subsequent cellulite formation.

- ❑ Stimulates formation of new bone tissue. Whereas estrogen promotes healthy bones by *decreasing* bone loss, progesterone does it by *increasing* bone growth.

- ❑ Helps prevent abnormal blood clotting.

- ❑ Has a calming effect on mood.

- ❑ Enhances the activity of thyroid hormone on energy production.

- ❑ Improves the sex drive.

- ❑ Helps stabilizes blood sugar.

- ❑ Contributes to a healthier LDL/HDL cholesterol ratio.

- ❑ Serves as a powerful antioxidant.

The list could go on. But you get the idea. This is an extremely important hormone.

The level of progesterone generally starts to decline when a woman reaches the mid thirties. Within a few years, the decline accelerates so significantly that it is deficient in every woman over the age of forty-five.

For all the reasons in the list above, the benefits of progesterone replacement in woman 35 and older can be truly remarkable.

Estrogen Dominance

A major progesterone role is to counteract "estrogen dominance." While many gynecologists ignore this issue, it is nonetheless pivotal when considering breast and uterine cancer, endometriosis, fibrocystic breast disease, PMS, cellulite, weight gain, and water retention. It is as big a problem with young women as with the older set.

A deficiency of progesterone is equivalent to an excess of estrogen. When this imbalance occurs it is referred to as estrogen dominance. The most common disorder occurring from estrogen dominance is PMS, with its symptoms of water retention, breast swelling, irritability, insomnia, depression, anxiety, loss of libido, and pelvic pain. This is low progesterone at work. In most cases it can be readily corrected by starting a progesterone replacement program.

Estrogen dominance is initially caused by a combination of decreased liver function and excessive environmental exposure to so-called "xenoestrogens."

Xenoestrogens

You may not have heard of them, but xenoestrogens are common synthetic chemicals that can act like human estrogens. These compounds are used commercially in solvents, pesticides, herbicides, fungicides, paper, and plastics. You can't escape them!

Over the years, xenoestrogens have thoroughly infiltrated the food chain. You probably didn't know it but you may be getting a barrage of these estrogen-like compounds every time you eat. Perhaps the greatest exposure is from beef, chicken, and pork that are routinely dosed up with estrogens in the feed lots.

Xenoestrogens are a major problem. They are believed to contribute to the modern day rise in both male and female sterility. Many researchers feel they are also behind the growing incidence of premature secondary sex characteristics so commonly seen in our children.

Suppressed Ovulation - More Common Than Realized

Ovulation occurs about ten days after the menstrual period begins. This triggers the production of progesterone. However, as xenoestrogens build up in the body, they can suppress normal ovulation, causing progesterone production to dramatically decrease. The result: estrogen dominance.

Traditionally, doctors have always thought that suppressed ovulation occurred only rarely in regularly menstruating women, but recent research shows that it is much more common than previously realized.

Birth control pills also suppress ovulation, and inasmuch as they contain strong synthetic estrogen compounds, they can rather drastically increase estrogen dominance.

As a result of aging, suppressed ovulation becomes even more commonplace in women as they approach their mid-forties. The ensuing estrogen dominance that develops causes cellulite and weight gain around the hips, and increases the risk of breast and uterine cancer.

Obviously, we should avoid the "-cides," and eat only hormone free beef, chicken, and pork whenever possible. Additionally, we shouldn't store foods in soft plastic wraps because they are a common source of xenoestrogens.

Another powerful strategy is QuickStart™, the supplement I developed and discussed in my Secret No. 5. This formula promotes detoxification and gives major nutritional support to the liver. Your liver is ultimately responsible for removing xenoestrogens from your system. It needs all the help you can give it.

Along with QuickStart™, a high fiber diet will do much to help the clean up process.

But My Doctor Says.....

Doctors often tell patients that a woman who has had a hysterectomy doesn't need progesterone replacement. I guess if a woman were simply a large uterus with legs the doctors would have a point. The truth is that such "logic" disregards all the many beneficial effects of progesterone I listed a moment ago, as well as ignores the fact that virtually every organ in a woman's body has progesterone receptor sites.

Let me state emphatically that every woman needs progesterone whether or not she has a uterus.

I believe this because the effects of estrogen dominance are so obvious in women whether or not they have had a hysterectomy. To one degree or another most women will have complaints of anxiety, irritability, insomnia, water retention, weight gain, cellulite, PMS, fatigue, menstrual pain or endometriosis, fibrocystic breasts, gall stones, uterine fibroids, blood clotting disorders, or migraines. These are symptoms or disorders caused by estrogen dominance, and likewise they can be successfully treated using natural hormonal replacement with progesterone.

Provera® is Not Progesterone

One more comment about progesterone, or specifically about a drug masquerading as progesterone. It's called medroxy-progesterone acetate, and it is commonly marketed as the patented drug Provera®. This is the product routinely prescribed by many doctors as a progesterone replacement.

If it were a real hormone, it would not be patentable. But, as a drug, it is patentable, and thus has been heavily promoted for years as a substitute for the real thing.

Make no mistake about it, although medroxy-progesterone acetate may be a pharmaceutical bestseller, it can be a real problem for the human body.

Like any physician, I am appreciative for many of the modern drugs developed by the pharmaceutical industry. These drugs literally save innumerable lives every day. But drugs should be properly used as therapeutic agents. They should not be prescribed as replacements for hormones, or for any other naturally occurring compound for that matter.

If you were to look at the Physicians' Desk Reference (PDR) and check out the common side effects of medroxy-progesterone acetate, you would wonder how doctors could prescribe it. The list reads like a who's who of side effects including: acne, rashes, weight gain, depression, breast tenderness, diabetes, head hair loss, facial hair growth, fluid retention, blood clots, pulmonary embolism, breast cancer, and birth defects.

That doesn't sound even remotely similar to what real progesterone does.

Why would anyone want to take this drug, or any other drug in this class of progesterone substitutes called "progestins," when real, natural progesterone is now readily available?

The answer is they take the drug because that's what their doctors prescribe. Many doctors are unaware of the natural option, or are not interested in it. And many patients, particularly those who are not up on the latest, don't know about natural progesterone.

I find that a topical progesterone cream works the best for the majority of my female patients. This is because oral progesterone often does not generate adequate tissue levels of the hormone. There are some excellent natural progesterone creams available over-the-counter. If you decide to use one of these creams, be sure to have your physician check your salivary progesterone level in order to be sure that you are taking the correct dose.

Thyroid: The "Master Hormones"

The thyroid gland is responsible for making your trillions of cells get to work. Your cells are like little factories. They take in oxygen, fat, carbohydrate, protein, and nutrients and from all these raw materials produce the energy along with specific peptides, steroids, enzymes, and saccharides that enable us to function.

The complex operation inside your cellular factories is called metabolism. Without adequate metabolism the cells will cease to work and you would cease to live! To keep this fundamental process running on full steam takes an adequate amount of the thyroid hormones, T3 and T4.

In the absence of adequate levels of the thyroid hormones, every single cell in your body will slow down. It's no wonder then that the symptoms associated with a malfunctioning thyroid read like a litany of what can go wrong in the human body.

The most common problem resulting from an aging thyroid gland is a lower production of thyroid hormone. The condition is called hypothyroidism. More than half of American men and women over 40 experience *three or more* symptoms related to hypothyroidism. And over the age of 50, I find that it is fairly uncommon to have an optimally functioning thyroid.

The thyroid gland, wrapped around the front of your windpipe just below the Adam's apple, produces these "master hormones." I call them "master hormones" for a very simple reason. **All the other hormones in your body are dependent on them for their own optimal function.** Even if you have optimal levels of other hormones, they will not work properly if T3 and T4 are deficient.

Broda Barnes, M.D., And The Myth Of The "Normal Thyroid"

Years ago, when I first began to study alternative medical treatments I read a book on the unrecognized prevalence of hypothyroidism and the importance of thyroid replacement. The book was written in 1976 by the late Broda Barnes, M.D., a veteran physician who practiced in the days when medicine was as much a clinical art as a science. He felt that an excellent way to determine the presence of a thyroid deficiency was to monitor the body temperature using a basal thermometer.

This is a simple enough procedure. So I began having patients take their underarm temperature when they awoke in the morning.

It didn't take long before I realized that probably no more than 5 percent of my patients had a normal reading. If Barnes was correct, the great majority of my patients needed thyroid replacement, despite the fact that almost all of them tested normal for thyroid using standard laboratory tests.

I was confused. To make matters even more confusing, Barnes said that the correct thyroid dose was one that restored the temperatures to an optimum level. But in order to accomplish this, I would have to give many patients doses of thyroid that were much higher than what was considered the maximum output of an adult thyroid.

I decided to try Barnes' approach. After all, it was based on thirty-five years of clinical experience with thousands of patients. Soon, my patients started telling me the same things that Barnes' patient had reported to him. They said they never felt so good in all their life, and that many long-standing and unresolved symptoms had vanished.

Apparently Barnes, the old master clinician, had discovered something very profound, and yet completely perplexing to me. How could so many patients do so well on thyroid doses that most experts would regard as excessive? And how was it possible that almost everyone I tested using the temperature test was found to have a low thyroid function?

It wasn't until almost twenty years later when I began using Bio-Energy Testing™ that I finally was able to answer these questions.

Why Do People Sometimes Need "Excessive" Thyroid Doses?

The answers lie beyond the thyroid itself, with the hypothalamus, a center within the brain that regulates the homeostatic control of the body, and with our old friend, the liver.

The hypothalamus is the hormone thermostat for the body. It is very sensitive to the body's need for thyroid hormone. When it senses that the body's metabolic rate is too slow, it sends a signal to the pituitary gland to release thyroid stimulating hormone (TSH). TSH then goes to the thyroid and stimulates it to make T4, an inactive form of the thyroid hormone. T4 then circulates through the blood stream to the liver where it is converted into T3, the active form of the hormone. It is T3 that is responsible for stimulating the cells to increase their metabolic rate, and thus keep the cells, tissues, and organs functioning properly.

The liver converts T4 to T3 on a "demand basis." When there is a greater need for stepped up metabolism - for example, to support increased activity such as exercise - the liver responds by converting more T4 into T3.

All this activity is "read" by the hypothalamus. It turns down or turns up the hormonal juices as necessary.

I believe that the reason some of my patients thrive on higher doses of thyroid is that there is a break down in one or more aspects of this axis. In many cases the problem may be a sluggish liver, in which case a revitalization of the liver will allow lower thyroid doses to be just as effective. In other cases, the problem may lie in the hypothalamus or the pituitary.

Why Does Almost Everyone Need Thyroid?

No one really knows exactly why the decline in the thyroid axis function is so common. Perhaps it is simply the effect of aging. After all, few things are more certain than the decline in metabolic rate associated with aging.

But thyroid axis decline can also develop from estrogen dominance, excessive fluoride supplementation, selenium and zinc deficiency, silver dental fillings (they contain mercury, that is highly toxic to the thyroid gland), and dental, chiropractic, and medical x-rays. These are commonplace factors, and may represent the real culprits behind thyroid underfunction.

Thyroid axis decline is much more common in women, even in young women, and I can't help but believe that estrogen dominance is the major factor for the decline. Conversely, a decline in thyroid activity results in a lack of ovulation in women, which in turn causes estrogen dominance. This vicious cycle is a particularly common one.

A Case of "Subclinical Hypothyroidism"

The heavy dependence that many doctors have on monitoring thyroid function through blood tests is a major problem in my opinion. The following case dramatizes my concern.

Loretta was 52-years-old and healthy according to her previous physician, despite the fact she had been complaining of tiredness, lack of energy, weight gain, dry skin, and cold intolerance for eight years. She also had an increasing cholesterol level.

She knew that her symptoms and her elevated cholesterol are commonly related to low thyroid function. Over the years she repeatedly asked her doctor to try a trial dose of thyroid hormone. Her doctor, however, was wedded to the thyroid blood tests. He refused her request because in all cases her results had been within the normal range.

She finally came to my clinic because she read an article I had written regarding the inaccuracy of conventional thyroid testing.

I checked her M-Factor by Bio-Energy Testing™ and was not at all surprised to find she was running at about 60 percent of optimum. Since she also had many symptoms of hypothyroidism, I started her on a trial of thyroid hormone replacement.

Loretta lived out of town, and called me in about four weeks.

"I feel like I have been given a second chance at life," she said, elatedly.

Her symptoms were gone. Her cholesterol readings had also much improved.

A couple of years went by before I heard from her again. It turns out she had sprained her ankle a few months before and had seen her regular doctor for treatment. When he learned she had been taking thyroid replacement, he became quite upset, insisting that all her tests failed to show the need for the hormone.

Loretta explained the results of her testing, but like many physicians he was unfamiliar with Bio-Energy Testing™. He took some blood tests again, which appeared to indicate that she did not need the thyroid she had been taking. He then insisted she discontinue the thyroid replacement or she would face risk of having too much thyroid.

Because of his insistence, she stopped taking the thyroid. Within two weeks she began to notice a return of her symptoms, and when she saw the doctor two months later she was back to feeling as bad as ever. In spite of this rather obvious clinical example of thyroid hormone deficiency, her physician still maintained she didn't need any replacement therapy because the "blood tests are all normal." He appeared to be happier having a miserable patient who had normal tests than a well patient on "too much thyroid."

It may seem strange to you, but many physicians are so devoted to laboratory test results that they often ignore what their patients are feeling. Needless to say, Loretta had had enough. She called my clinic, and was restarted on the hormone replacement that she so obviously needed.

Bio-Energy Testing™ To The Rescue

Loretta was smart enough to listen to her body. But many other people are relegated to permanent misery simply because they have what is described in the medical literature as "sub-clinical hypothyroidism."

This means patients who have low thyroid function in the face of lab results that fall within the normal range. A 1983 study published in *Postgraduate Medicine* covered this issue. It was entitled, "How to detect hypothyroidism when screening tests are normal."

In the study, sixty-five women, like Loretta, were examined because their many symptoms were suggestive of hypothyroidism. In all cases, the blood tests were within normal range. Using a sophisticated stimulation challenge test, the researchers demonstrated that forty-seven of the women, or 72 percent, did in fact have hypothyroidism despite the normal tests.

Guess what happened when they were treated with thyroid hormone? They improved!

Various studies have revealed that in any given age group somewhere between 5-15 percent of the population has hypothyroidism despite normal thyroid blood tests.

One of the great advantages of Bio-Energy Testing™ is that it is the most sensitive way to determine the presence of low thyroid function, and even subclinical hypothyroidism. Low thyroid function is indicated by a low M-Factor.

Testosterone

Testosterone is considered the male sex hormone. But it's not a man's thing exclusively. Women make a bit as well, a small, but important amount that greatly contributes to their health. Deficiency in females leads to diminished or lost sex drive, depression, apathy, joint aches and pains, fat gain, loss of exercise endurance, and osteoporosis. Deficiency is almost always present in women who have had a hysterectomy.

But back to the men.

Unlike women, who have been studied for sex hormone deficiency for decades, male testosterone deficiency has been largely ignored in this country. Unlike the rapid decline of sex hormones experienced by women, the loss of testosterone in men is often quite slow, gradually taking effect over ten to fifteen years. Because the decline in function occurs so slowly, men seldom fully realize the nature of what has happened to them.

Another reason why men just haven't gotten "equal treatment" is related to the male ego, and the "nothing is wrong" mentality.

I routinely see this attitude among my male patients. Sometimes it is almost comical. Let me give you a typical example of an interview in my office with a 55 or 60-year-old man.

Me: "So how's your sex life?"

Him: "Not a problem."

Me: "O.K., how about your memory."

Him: "Not a problem."

Me: "Great. How about your moods?"

Him: "Seems fine."

Me: "And how's your strength and stamina?"

Him: "No complaints there either, Doc."

Me: "O.K. Now I want you to compare how all these things are to how they were ten or fifteen years ago."

He thinks for a few moments.

"Of course, I'm not the man I used to be," he admits. "Those were the days. Nothing could get me down! I could have sex all the time, stay out all night long, and get up in the morning and........"

It's often only when men really honestly compare their current level of function to that of their "peak" years that they realize there has been a definite decline.

Grumpy Old Men

Few things in medicine are as rewarding to me as replacing a depleted man's testosterone. Few things seem to be as rewarding to the man's wife as well.

I vividly remember the time I walked into the clinic one morning and saw a gorgeous arrangement of roses on the counter.

Being a big lover of flowers, I immediately asked, "Well, who did what to get those?" The answer from the staff was, "That's what we'd like to know. They're for you."

The card was from one of my women patients and read as follows:

"Roses are red,

"Violets are blue,

"My husband's a stud,

"All thanks to you!"

It wasn't just his renewed interest in sex, a result of testosterone replacement, that had this lady so pleased. It was also his remarkable improvement in mood.

Testosterone has a marked uplifting effect on the mood of both men and women. The positive enthusiasm, passion, and risk-taking characteristics of men are mediated by testosterone. As men age and their testosterone levels decrease, they tend to become grumpy, irritable, apathetic, and listless.

Tiberius Reiter, M.D., first reported the benefits of testosterone replacement for men back in the early 1960s. After twelve years, and two hundred and forty patients who complained of premature aging, he described the following results: "Men who were stooped, slow moving, slow thinking, and considering retirement like old men came back for a check-up at two months looking quite different. They walk well, hold themselves erect, and talk and act like very young 50 year olds instead of very old 60 year olds. There is even a change in the voice, manner, and handshake."

Testosterone And Your Heart

It's a connection that nobody ever makes: testosterone and the heart.

The fact is that testosterone exerts great protective and therapeutic effects on the heart. This shouldn't be too strange because after all, the heart is a muscle, and testosterone exerts a powerful effect on muscle function. The benefit is particularly significant for diabetics, but also applies to *all* men and women with heart disease.

Testosterone deficiency causes an undesirable decrease in the HDL/LDL cholesterol ratio associated with atherosclerosis. In addition, it contributes to elevated triglycerides, insulin resistance, elevated blood pressure, coronary artery blockage, and increased tendency for blood clotting.

Testosterone replacement reverses these negative developments. Patients report improvements on many fronts: cardiac function, treadmill testing, chest pain, weight management, lipid profile, blood clotting, and glucose control.

Men - and women as well - with heart disease should definitely explore testosterone replacement therapy.

Testosterone and Your Prostate

Many doctors shy away from testosterone replacement, fearing it will aggravate the prostate. This fear persists despite the reality that both prostate cancer and prostate enlargement only develop in older men with lower testosterone levels.

I carefully monitor the prostate status of all my patients on testosterone replacement, just as I routinely do with all my elderly male patients. The only effect on the prostate from proper testosterone replacement therapy that I have seen is *uniform improvement*. PSA, a blood test commonly used to diagnose the early stages of prostate cancer, almost always improve. Bladder function improves.

I rarely see the opposite occur. Perhaps this is because I also carefully monitor the estrogen level.

Women have some testosterone. And yes, men have some estrogen.

In men the enzyme aromatase converts testosterone to estrogen. For reasons that are not fully known, this enzyme develops more activity as men age, resulting in higher levels of estrogen. If the estrogen levels get high enough, they will impair sexual function and desire. Additionally, it is elevated levels of estrogen in men that in all likelihood has more to do with prostate disorders than does testosterone.

Because of aromatase, testosterone replacement may stimulate an increase in estrogen levels in men. When this unpleasant complication occurs, it can be easily treated by optimizing liver function and taking an extract of the passion flower plant. This plant has the ability to block the activity of aromatase, and thus decrease elevated estrogen levels.

Another important concept regarding testosterone conversion to estrogen in men has to do with how the testosterone is administered. **While testosterone injections are notorious for causing this problem, testosterone creams and implants are much less likely to have this effect.**

In the 1996 book *"Maximizing Manhood,"* British physician Malcolm Carruthers describes his experience in treating more than a thousand men with testosterone replacement. He writes that after a half-century of treatment for hypogonadal patients with testosterone implants and thirty years of treatment with injections of testosterone there is no evidence of any associated rise in prostate cancer or even of benign prostatic hypertrophy.

Most researchers agree that properly administered testosterone replacement does not cause prostate cancer. However, men *who already have prostate cancer* need to know that testosterone replacement might induce the cancer to grow at an accelerated rate. With this in mind, I do not administer testosterone to male patients with prostate cancer, and only very cautiously to men with an elevated PSA.

As an additional precaution, all men supplemented with testosterone should receive annual digital prostate examinations along with PSA evaluations.

The Amazing Human Growth Hormone

The longer I use human growth hormone (HGH) replacement the more amazed I am. More so than any other hormone, HGH has the most wide-ranging and stunning anti-aging properties. It significantly influences virtually all aspects of aging, including the production of other hormones.

According to Daniel Rudman, M.D., the pioneering physician who first examined the effects of growth hormone replacement in aged men, "The overall deterioration of the body that comes with growing old is not inevitable. We now realize that some aspects of it can be prevented or reversed."

In an article published in 2000 in *Hormone Research*, the author concludes that life without growth hormone is poor in quality and quantity, and further makes the point that the usual growth hormone level of men in their sixties is *"indistinguishable" from patients with documented diseases of the pituitary gland.*

The only limitation to the use of growth hormone has been the cost factor. Just a few years ago, a month's supply of HGH would cost you $10,000.

Thanks to recombinant DNA technology and the fact that the patents on growth hormone have run out, the hormone can now be produced at a much more accessible level to meet the growing interest and demand. Today, a month's supply costs about $200.

HGH is named after the growth spurt synonymous with the teenage years. An enormous increase of HGH sparks this high-growth period. During this time of life, HGH blood levels can soar to as much as 2,000 mcg/L per day.

What goes up, must come down. Thus, after the sharp rise during the growth spurt, there is a sharp fall off. The average amount of HGH produced at age twenty is about 600 mcg/l. At thirty, about 400 mcg/l. By forty, the level is down to 250 mcg/l. And from here it tends to very slowly decrease over the next forty years to a lowly average of 25 mcg/l per day in 70 year olds.

The elevated level we see in the teenage years drives the growth spurt. The lower levels in adulthood serve to maintain that growth.

By the time you reach your fifties and your HGH levels are sagging below 200 mcg/l your body will also begin to sag - and shrink - as well. Ever so slowly. That's right. Your heart, lungs, brain, liver, and all the rest, actually reduce in size.

We refer to this downsizing as atrophy. You see it most noticeably as sagging muscles and skin. And you feel it most noticeably in the form of diminished function. You feel it in these ways:

❑ As the brain shrinks, you are not able to think as quickly and as clearly as you once could.

❑ As the heart atrophies, you won't have the stamina and endurance that you had.

❑ As the bones atrophy, you develop osteoporosis and become shorter.

❑ As the immune system atrophies, your resistance will suffer and you are more likely to develop infectious illnesses and cancer.

❑ As the hormone producing glands atrophy, you will have lower and lower levels of hormones.

HGH can slow down such central losses and even reverse the process in many cases, as the box on the next page indicates.

When To Start HGH

The original studies on HGH were performed on men aged seventy to seventy-two. As a result, many physicians and patients regard this general period as the appropriate time to start HGH replacement.

But more recent data indicates that the optimum time to start is much earlier. And it makes sense. Why start HGH therapy after all the "damage" has been done? Early physical signs of growth hormone deficiency include skeletal muscle loss as evidenced by sagging skin in the face, arms, and buttocks.

These signs are normally seen as we enter the fifties, and are often pronounced by the time we reach sixty. The laboratory blood test known as IGF-1 is an excellent indicator of your level of growth hormone. Optimum levels of IGF-1 should be greater than 200 ng/ml.

My IGF-1 levels dipped all the way down to 54 ng/ml when I was fifty-three. I was just starting to experience some of the signs and symptoms of growth hormone deficiency at the time, so I was not all that surprised. I have been on growth hormone replacement ever since, and literally all of the problems I was experiencing are now completely gone, and I feel and function as well as I did in my 30's. My current IGF-1 level is maintained at 300 ng/ml.

Documented Benefits Of HGH Therapy

- ❏ An 8.8 percent increase in muscle mass in 6 months without exercise.
- ❏ A 14.4 percent loss of fat mass in 6 months without dieting.
- ❏ Higher energy levels.
- ❏ Enhanced sexual performance.
- ❏ Re-growth of shrunken organs.
- ❏ Improved cardiac output.
- ❏ Improved immune function.
- ❏ Improved brain function.
- ❏ Improved sleep.
- ❏ Improved vision.
- ❏ Improved cholesterol parameters.
- ❏ Lowered blood pressure.
- ❏ Stronger bones.
- ❏ Faster healing.
- ❏ Tighter, thicker, more hydrated skin.
- ❏ Wrinkle reduction
- ❏ Hair re-growth.
- ❏ Cellulite reduction
- ❏ Mood elevation.
- ❏ PLUS: Enhancement of effects generated by replacement of other hormones.

The Case Of Robert's Knees

When Robert first saw me he was 62-years-old. Years of hard living had had both good and bad effects. He had been a hard drinker until he was fifty-five at which time he realized he had a problem. And he stopped.

"I've never been happier in my whole life than I have been since I stopped drinking," he told me. "The older I got the more I realized how important my kids are to me, and the drinking was just ruining my relationships."

On the good side of the equation was the fact that he had been a rancher all his life, and had always eaten real food, and spent hours each day doing hard work.

Robert appeared thin, well muscled for his age, but about ten years older than his stated age. All the years of drinking had definitely accelerated the aging process

He complained of moodiness, lack of sex drive, and insomnia, and further stated that he just did not have the energy to work around the ranch like he used to. He was only sleeping 5-6 hours "on a good night," but his major concern was his knees.

"An orthopedist told me my knees had been so deteriorated over the years from arthritis and hard work that the only solution available was joint replacement," he said.

Indeed, as he struggled to get out of the waiting room chair and slowly walked into my office, it was apparent that his knees were a serious impediment.

Robert's symptoms were so characteristic of testosterone deficiency that I did not even wait to get the tests back before starting him on replacement therapy. He was also started on QuickStart™, DHEA, lipoic acid, and a low dose of thyroid. I also made sure he was following all the other important steps outlined in this book.

When he returned six weeks later to go over the test results, he was already starting to notice more energy, but his other symptoms were still very present. The tests revealed that he was grossly deficient in growth hormone, and after I explained to him the many beneficial effects of HGH, he agreed to give it a try.

Two months later, on a return visit, he told me that his energy level is "starting to get much closer to the way it has always been, and best of all I am starting to really sleep well." He also said that his knees were starting to feel better. I noted that he was able to get out of the chair much more quickly.

Six months later, after a total of nine months on the program, he came back again and happily gave me the good news.

"I'm feeling as good as I ever have in my life, maybe even better," he said.

His knees were almost back to complete function. He was walking normally, and able to hike up hills he had not been able to even consider for years.

Robert's case is an excellent example of two important effects of HGH replacement. First, many of the beneficial effects of testosterone and DHEA replacement will simply not occur in the absence of adequate growth hormone replacement. Testosterone is a hormone that requires growth hormone to be present in order to really be effective.

Secondly, growth hormone can literally regenerate the lost cartilage in joints damaged by years of osteoarthritis and wear and tear.

The effects of HGH are mediated primarily through the action of the liver. For this reason, I recommend that anyone using HGH be sure to also include all the vitamins, minerals, and herbal supplements found in "QuickStart™." Along with the other steps in this book, they will guarantee optimal liver function.

In some cases I also recommend HGH "stimulators," namely certain amino acids that promote pituitary secretion of HGH. It must be noted, however, that the response to these stimulators is modest and quite variable, and as a rule these agents usually have no significant effect in the over fifty age group.

You will probably see and hear advertising of various brands of so-called "homeopathic" growth hormone products sold on the Internet and in stores. These products, often sold as capsules and sublingual sprays, purport to have growth hormone in them. Avoid them! Other than the placebo effect, I believe they are essentially worthless. All medical studies showing benefits from HGH therapy have involved the injectable form of the hormone. This is what I prescribe for interested patients.

Melatonin: More Than Just For Sleeping

We've all pretty much heard about this celebrated hormone as a result of front cover magazine treatment and the 1995 bestseller, *"The Melatonin Miracle."* Most people think of melatonin as a sleeping and jet lag aid. And indeed it helps for both. However, its benefits are much broader. Let me cover a bit of the sleep connection first and then move on to the other exciting effects of melatonin.

Studies have shown a consistent and progressive decline in melatonin production starting in the early twenties. By age fifty, your melatonin level is half of what it was in your early adult years. By seventy, it is less than half of what you had at fifty, and so on and so on, in a continuing decline.

Insomnia associated with aging? That's often a direct effect of ebbing melatonin. Twenty-year-olds sleep an average of ten hours a night. Sixty-year-olds only get in six hours or so of sleep, much of it restless.

In 1994, one of the first scientific studies reporting this effect was published in the *British Medical Journal*. The researchers demonstrated a direct relationship between the amount of melatonin being produced and the quality of sleep. They concluded that melatonin deficiency seems to be a key factor in the sleep disorders of the elderly.

Melatonin turns out to be a key element in the induction of a sleep cycle known as "slow wave sleep." **Slow wave sleep is the restorative stage of sleep**. This is when the body repairs the damage that has occurred during the day.

Ever wonder why someone over fifty doesn't heal as well from the stresses and strains of exercise or injury as they did when they were younger? You can blame much of that on a decreased level of melatonin. Austrian researchers have found that people who take a melatonin supplement spend a much longer time in slow wave sleep than those who do not.

It is interesting to note that the pituitary releases HGH during the slow wave stage of sleep. A recent study published in the *Journal of the American Medical Association* revealed that sleep deprivation resulted in significantly lowered levels of growth hormone production. This once again points out the close relationships between hormones.

But let's go beyond the melatonin-sleeping connection, which is really only the tip of the iceberg, and discover some of the other "talents" of this extremely important hormone.

We've Got Rhythm

Melatonin is a major player - perhaps *the* major player - in our natural biological cycle known as the circadian rhythm. It is this inner rhythm that acts like a biological clock, controlling our sleep/wake cycle, hormone and brain neurotransmitter production, body temperature, blood pressure, weight gain/loss, mood, energy level, and immunity.

Melatonin is secreted in a part of the brain behind your forehead known as the pineal gland. This gland is extremely sensitive to sunlight, and releases melatonin in direct relationship to our sunlight exposure. I've covered the importance of obtaining adequate sunlight in Secret No. 3. Now you have another reason for getting enough sun into your life. And, of course, getting enough sleep, which melatonin supplementation can enhance.

Our natural circadian rhythm is central to our biological functioning. Walter Pierpaoli, M.D., the world-famous Italian researcher, in a series of dramatic and elaborate laboratory experiments, demonstrated this fact in the early 1990s.

Working with Vladimir Lesnikov, Ph.D., a Russian researcher, Pierpaoli surgically exchanged the pineal glands of young mice with those of old mice. The rodents were genetically identical, thus there was no rejection of the transplants.

As expected, the younger mice with the old pineal glands soon began to show the unmistakable signs of accelerated aging. Meanwhile, the older mice with the transplanted young glands appeared rejuvenated.

At the end of the experiment, the "old" mice ended up living twice as long as the "young" ones!

In terms of human years, the "old" mice with the young glands lived over one hundred years. These experiments have led many experts in longevity medicine to regard melatonin as something of a fountain of youth.

Priming The Immune System

Melatonin also exerts a marked effect on the immune system. Studies have shown it can help in the treatment and prevention of breast and prostate cancer.

Melatonin appears to enhance the immune activity of the thymus gland, located in the upper chest just below the neck. The thymus is a repository of first-line immune cells called lymphocytes. And it is here, in this gland, that immature lymphocytes go through a conditioning process - sort of like immune system "boot camp" - that turns them into disease-fighting units that protect your body.

Alas, as we age, the thymus gland also atrophies and increasingly loses its ability to produce mature immune cells called T-lymphocytes. This results in the lowered immune response so common in the elderly.

Receptor sites for melatonin have been found both on thymus cells and lymphocytes. In 1993, European researcher George Maestroni published the first study demonstrating that melatonin stimulated the production of T-lymphocytes in persons with lowered immune function. He concluded that "the pineal gland might thus be viewed as the crux of a sophisticated immuno-neuroendocrine network."

Melatonin The Antioxidant

Melatonin also provides another major benefit to the body: as an antioxidant. As I have mentioned before in this book, free radicals create much, if not most, of the deterioration that occurs in the body as we age. Crucial antioxidant vitamins such as vitamin C and E, along with CoQ10, are primary agents that snuff out free radical activity.

Melatonin, as an antioxidant, possesses its very own unique ability. An article written by melatonin researcher R. Hardeland concluded that melatonin is an even more potent antioxidant than both vitamins C and E.

Additionally, researchers have also discovered that melatonin penetrates all the way into the nucleus of cells, where its antioxidant activity protects DNA from the type of free radical destruction that can lead to cancer and neurological disease.

It is thought that melatonin may be able to limit the incidence of memory loss, Alzheimer's, and other brain disorders so common to the elderly.

Ray Sahelian, M.D., author of an excellent book on melatonin entitled *Melatonin, Nature's Sleeping Pill*, says that taken as a supplement, melatonin "could slow down the aging process and decrease the incidences of brain damage and cancer."

I recommend starting melatonin supplementation around the age of forty-five. This is when your body's production has started to go downhill. Try a small dose at first. I find that very little (such as half a milligram) is needed to maintain a youthful level. Even though melatonin in very high doses has been shown to be non-toxic, I find that occasionally patients will develop sleep disturbances and morning drowsiness when they take more than they need. Melatonin should be taken about one half an hour before bedtime.

DHEA

Of all the hormones supplemented for anti-aging reasons, DHEA is perhaps the best known. A lot has been written and said about it. Just to get it out of the way - and never bring it up again (you will no doubt be relieved) - DHEA stands for dehydroepiandrosterone.

Considerable research has been conducted showing that low levels of this adrenal hormone are associated with virtually every disease studied. The list includes cardiovascular disease, cancer, diabetes, osteoporosis, Alzheimer's, lupus, AIDS, and viral and bacterial infections.

Clinically, I don't see the obvious and immediate clinical benefit from DHEA replacement that I observe routinely with HGH, estrogen, progesterone, and testosterone therapy. The effects of these other hormones are often more dramatic than those of DHEA. Nevertheless, I regard DHEA as an extremely important element in a total disease prevention strategy.

DHEA is the most abundant steroid hormone in the body and is secreted in response to virtually any kind of stress. By age seventy-five, however, you only produce about 10 percent of the amount you could make as a 25-year-old.

DHEA has been labeled as the "mother" of all hormones. That's because it can, and often is, converted by the body into estrogen compounds and testosterone. The conversion rate differs widely among individuals but is significant enough so that anyone taking DHEA needs to have these other hormones monitored.

Many human studies involving DHEA supplementation report that most patients experience a feeling of "well being." I have also found this generalized rejuvenation effect to be very consistent in my patients as well.

I also see my elderly patients on DHEA recovering much more quickly from flu and colds. Only rarely do these infections last beyond a mild three or four day illness.

This is attributable in part to the ability of DHEA to boost the immune response in older people. Animal studies have shown that DHEA protects the thymus gland from the "normal" shrinking that is associated with aging. This is the same thymus gland that I mentioned a moment ago in relation to melatonin. So here is another hormone that is "thymus-friendly."

Other promising animal studies have shown regression of tumors when animals were supplemented with DHEA.

My Recommendations:

❑ *If you are over forty*, look for a physician familiar with natural hormonal testing and replacement therapy. He or she can gently and safely "escort" you into an effective program that will revitalize your life. *Do it now, even if you feel great! Remember, the best treatment is prevention.* Don't wait to be symptomatic.

❑ You can find a referral for an experienced physician near you by visiting the American Academy of Anti-Aging Medicine's web site at www.worldhealth.net, or calling the organization at (719) 475-8775.

❑ Use Bio-Energy Testing™ to determine if your M-Factor is abnormally low. If it is, be sure your hormone replacement program includes thyroid. Don't rely on a thyroid blood test alone to monitor your replacement dosage. These tests miss low thyroid states in a great many cases. That's why a Bio-Energy Testing™ analysis is the best way to go. You can obtain a referral to a Bio-Energy Testing™ certified health care practitioner in your area by visiting my web site at www.bursting-with-energy.com, or by calling 1-866-376-0610. Remember also that the hallmark of aging is a decreased E.Q. as determined by Bio-Energy Testing™. So be sure that no matter how great you feel, your program optimizes your E.Q.!

❑ Many natural hormones are available over the counter or through the Internet. However, I always discourage people from getting their hormones this way. Many products are ineffective and some do not contain the potency they claim to contain. *For hormones, a trained medical physician is really necessary.* And through the doctor, and the compounding pharmacy he or she uses, you can purchase the very best quality of natural hormones.

Secret No. 9
Weight Control And Energy

According to government statistics, more than 60 percent of American adults are overweight. One-quarter are classified as obese, putting them at increased risk for chronic diseases such as heart disease, diabetes, high blood pressure, stroke, and some forms of cancer. And, very sad to say, our children are following suit. A weight problem among youngsters is now at an epidemic level.

By all accounts, we appear to be the most obese people in the world, and growing more so every year.

Obesity is not just an appearance problem. It is a profound health problem. It is by far the single major statistical risk factor for developing serious diseases. Medical experts say it is an independent or aggravating agent for more than thirty medical conditions.

You just can't be healthy and obese at the same time.

There are many reasons for obesity, including bad eating habits, a stressful and sedentary lifestyle, improper exercise, inadequate sleep, and age related hormonal and nutritional deficiencies.

Maintaining one's weight at a proper and healthy level is obviously a major element in physical and emotional wellness. And for many people it's a major lifetime struggle, involving the challenge of replacing habits that aren't working with new habits that do. **Habits are difficult to break, but it can be done if the *will and desire* is strong enough.** The good news is that once you develop new habits they will be just as hard to break as the old ones.

The rewards are impressive. Healthy weight pays off in terms of a healthier, happier life...and a longer life as well.

In this chapter I would like to offer a *different approach to weight loss.* It is an approach based on years of guiding frustrated patients with resistant weight problems to a more normal and healthier weight. If you are such a person, the information here can help you reach this critical and elusive health goal.

Are You Too Heavy?

Most of us can easily tell if we have too much fat simply by looking in the mirror. But a more exact way of assessing obesity is often needed. For sure, your fat stores cannot be objectively measured simply by checking your weight. Your total weight, what you see on the scale, is a mixture of your muscle weight and your fat weight. As you will see, muscle weight cancels out the negative effects of fat weight to such an extent that saying an individual has too much body fat is basically the same as saying they have too little muscle.

You might wonder how professional football players who have so much obvious fat can still be so quick and powerful. The answer of course is that underneath the fat is a huge amount of muscle that is not so obvious to the eye.

Heaviness - "Officially Defined"

The National Institute of Diabetes and Digestive and Kidney Diseases of the National Institutes of Health is the lead federal agency responsible for biomedical research on obesity.

From this resource, we have the following "official" definitions:"

❑ **Overweight**

An excess amount of body weight that includes muscle, bone, fat, and water.

❑ **Obesity**

To most people, the term "obesity" means to be very overweight. But "obesity" specifically refers to an excess amount of body fat. Some people, such as bodybuilders or other athletes with a lot of muscle, can be overweight without being obese.

Everyone needs a certain amount of body fat for stored energy, cold insulation, and other functions. As a rule, women have more body fat than men. Most health care providers agree that men with more than 25 percent body fat and women with more than 30 percent body fat are obese.

One of the best ways to determine how much fat and muscle weight you have is by using an electronic technique called bio-impedance measurement. Bio-impedance testing is quick, safe, easy, and readily available in fitness centers and from anti-aging physicians. It involves passing a small level of electrical current through the body. Since muscle and fat each conduct current in different ways, it is possible to determine how much of each is present.

Ideal body fat measurements are 12 to 18 percent for men and 18 to 22 percent for women. Without pulling any punches, let me say that to the degree that your body fat measurement is greater than this, you are unhealthy, and will develop diseases that are otherwise completely preventable.

Obesity = Energy Deficit

There is no more obvious a disorder of energy balance than obesity.

And perhaps the most important point regarding obesity and energy production relates to fat metabolism. **Specifically, every time we eat a meal, the energy from that meal is stored as fat. It doesn't make any difference whether the meal is carbohydrate or fat. Practically speaking, *it all gets stored as fat.***

This is how Nature designed it.

As I have said before, you need to remember that we have evolved over many thousands of years. In the distant past, our ancestors were never quite sure when the next meal was coming. Only recently in our evolutionary development has the concept of three meals a day become commonplace for many humans. Yet the timeless physiological process of storing meals as fat has not changed.

The fat stored from your meal is meant to serve your energy requirements until the next one. But what if your body's ability to produce energy from this stored fat is impaired? In this case, you will not only gain weight because you can't break down your fat stores, but you will also produce less energy as well. **The two go hand in hand. Gaining weight and having low energy are two sides of the same coin - an inability to burn or metabolize fat**. This is a very common scenario as we get older, and is also why people are unable to lose weight.

All obese individuals, with the exception of the few who just eat too much, have a serious flaw in the ability to produce energy efficiently. Without measuring energy production and correcting the underlying disorders of energy production it becomes almost impossible to permanently correct obesity.

That's the theory. Here are the facts:

- ❑ 75 percent of all persons who lose weight regain it within three years.

- ❑ 95 percent regain it within ten years.

Why were the 5 percent who initially lost weight able to keep it off? No doubt because they somehow managed to correct the energy production deficit that caused their obesity in the first place.

Low energy production causes obesity.

And obesity causes low energy production.

Many patients fall into such a deep hole from this vicious cycle that it appears impossible for them to escape. What initiates this vicious cycle in the first place?

Too Much Insulin

The answer, and the first step towards obesity, involves a loss in energy production resulting from a condition known as "insulin resistance." Before explaining what this means let me take a moment to give you a brief backgrounder.

Our DNA, tissues, and organs are made entirely of fat, protein, and minerals. We consume these raw materials in our food. The body extracts them from food in the digestive process, and after they are processed in the liver, uses them as needed.

We also consume carbohydrates. But nothing in the body is made of carbohydrates.

The body extracts vitamins and minerals from the carbohydrates and puts them to use in the body. The fiber contained in the carbohydrates, assuming that it has not been processed out, such as in refined sugars and grains, is used by the body as roughage to promote elimination of waste products and other toxins.

The absorbed sugars, extracted from the carbohydrates, represent a raw material for energy production. But the reality is that the body can make all the energy it needs from fat alone.

When we consume carbohydrates, the body does one or two things with the extracted sugars: burns them for energy, or stores them as fat. The decision to burn or store is primarily determined by hormones. And the most important hormone in this scenario is insulin, secreted by the pancreas according to the amount of carbohydrate in your diet.

The connection between carbohydrate consumption and obesity is this: The more carbohydrates you eat, the more insulin the pancreas makes. Obesity is often caused by the presence of too much insulin.

Insulin diverts ingested carbohydrates to fat storage and away from energy production. So it is easy to see why excess insulin creates a low energy state combined with increased body fat.

And here's the rest of the story:

Another function of insulin is to prevent the breakdown and utilization of stored fat.

As I explained in Chapter 3, outside of exercise, a hormonally balanced individual produces his or her energy almost completely from stored fat. However, since insulin prevents the breakdown and utilization of fat, you can see that in a state of insulin excess you would have to get a majority of your energy from stored carbohydrate, known as glycogen. The significant difference between glycogen and fat stores is that the former is used up rapidly. Glycogen can usually provide energy for only one or two hours. By comparison, fat stores can provide energy for days and even weeks.

In a state of insulin excess, the following happens:

1. **In only a few hours after eating, after your glycogen stores are depleted, you will begin to run out of energy, a state known as hypoglycemia, or low blood sugar.**

2. **You will have a persistent craving for carbohydrate to replenish the exhausted glycogen stores.**

The Insulin/Carbohydrate Vicious Cycle

Succumbing to the craving sets up the vicious cycle. Eating more carbs stimulates the body to make more insulin. The more insulin you make, the more difficult it is for your body to access fat for energy, and so you readily use up your glycogen stores. The more you use up your glycogen stores, the more you need to eat carbohydrate. Ad infinitum.

The nasty effects of this cycle stem from the resultant decrease in energy production, and include fatigue, headaches, depression, anxiety, and insomnia. Another very common effect is a persistent weight gain that you will not be able to lose even when you exercise and limit caloric intake. Let me repeat. **IN A STATE OF INSULIN EXCESS, YOU WILL NOT BE ABLE TO LOSE WEIGHT EVEN IF YOU EXERCISE AND LIMIT CALORIES UNTIL YOU ARE BLUE IN THE FACE!!**

A moment ago I said the first step towards obesity is a decrease in energy production from insulin resistance. Insulin resistance refers to the decreased ability of the body's cells to respond to insulin. That is, they become resistant to the hormone, a predicament caused by a combination of genetics, hormonal deficiencies, multiple nutrient deficiencies (especially fatty acids and chromium), stress, insomnia, and too sedentary a lifestyle.

When the body's cells become resistant to insulin, the pancreas responds by making more insulin. Another vicious cycle is created.

As insulin resistance continues over years, the pancreas keeps pumping out ever increasing amounts of insulin. Ultimately a state of chronic insulin excess develops. And by blocking the utilization of fat stores for energy production, the constantly elevated insulin levels eventually result in the excessive fat stores we refer to as obesity.

As this situation continues, the fat cells themselves become progressively larger (the fat cells become fatter!). They expand to such an extent that the insulin receptor sites on the membranes become stretched and distorted, and unable to properly respond to insulin. In other words, these engorged fat cells become resistant to insulin, which in turn acts to further increase the already elevated insulin levels.

How Obesity Causes Low Energy

There's still more to this drama of vicious cycles, and particularly how obesity, in turn, causes low energy. I personally believe that the low energy state comes first, but this is pretty much of a mute point. The reality is that when most people become concerned about their weight, both factors are in full force: low energy production and obesity.

Obesity results in low energy production in a number of ways:

❑ First, obesity leads to decreased muscle mass. This is no doubt a result of the decreased levels of activity and exercise so commonly seen in obese persons. However, decreased muscle mass is also a side effect of the hormonal deficiencies that helped to cause the obesity in the first place. Since muscle mass is such metabolically active tissue, any decrease in muscle mass only serves to further lower the metabolic rate, which typically results in more fat gain. This is measured by the Bio-Energy Testing™ analyzer as an abnormally low M-Factor.

❑ Secondly, obesity causes a variety of sleep disturbances. These disturbances are often manifested by snoring and daytime sleepiness, but frequently they are present without symptoms, and can only be detected in a sleep lab.

An extremely common problem with obesity is that it interferes with the body's ability to enter into what is known as the "slow wave" stage of sleep. You might remember that I discussed the importance of slow wave sleep in the section on melatonin. Since the majority of growth hormone production occurs during slow wave sleep, this leads to a deficiency of growth hormone. You might remember that the hallmark of growth hormone deficiency is a decrease in muscle mass and an increase in fat mass.

The sleep disturbances associated with obesity also create more insulin resistance. How this occurs is still unknown, but the fact that it happens is well documented.

❑ Obesity also causes an excess of estrogens. This is because fat cells metabolically increase estrogens in the body independent of ovarian and adrenal gland production. In excess, estrogens suppress mitochondria, resulting in a significant reduction in metabolism. Estrogens also cause the body to retain and increase fat stores. You see the result as unsightly cellulite.

Note to the men: Excess estrogens also affect you, because you produce estrogens in the adrenal glands, and as you age a greater proportion of your testosterone becomes converted to estrogen. This not only causes fat gain, but can also contribute to prostate enlargement as well as prostate cancer.

❑ Obese persons engage in much less physical activity. A sedentary lifestyle translates to a lower metabolic rate. Often, obese individuals are exercise intolerant. As I noted in the chapter on exercise, they can easily slip into anaerobic energy production that makes exercising effectively very difficult.

Other Weight Control Aggravators

The factors I have mentioned thus far form the basis for most of the weight control problems for obese individuals. There are still several others that can stymie a weight loss effort.

One is sunlight deficiency. Several studies examining the effects of sunlight deficiency have demonstrated a significant association with a lowered metabolic rate in both animals and humans. This occurs as a result of hormonal deficiencies created by a lack of sunlight plus other as yet unidentified effect(s) of sunlight deprivation.

Stress is another cause of decreased metabolism. In a majority of individuals, prolonged stress decreases the metabolic rate through its negative impact on the output of the adrenal glands, leading to low blood sugar, low energy production, and weight gain.

Inadequate water intake depresses the metabolism. Dehydration can lead to overeating because it often causes the feeling of hunger.

Insomnia and lack of adequate rest can also lower the metabolic rate.

And then there is the issue of emotional eating. **In our overfed society, much of what we consider hunger often has more to do with emotions than with real physical need**. In this regard I believe *that all of us,* thin and overweight alike, have an eating disorder to some extent. Periodic fasting (see Chapter 4) can help you identify how much of a reality this might be for you.

Training yourself to be comfortable and relaxed when you are hungry is a major step to solving the problem of emotional eating. An invaluable technique to help you attain this ability is to fast once a week, and use the breath meditation exercise when you feel hungry. This won't lessen your feeling of hunger, but it will help you to control all the emotions that hunger stirs up.

Metabolic Weight Loss

If you have a serious weight problem, you now know the possible reasons for it.

What's next is to lose the fat. And to do that permanently you must normalize your energy production. You must make that a primary goal.

This means optimizing your M-Factor and your E and Q.

How Much Fat Do You Lose While You're Sleeping?

Your energy production level at rest, i.e., when you are sleeping, is referred to as your basal metabolism. A therapeutic tenet of the Energy Deficit Theory of aging is that no matter what age you are or what genetics you've been dealt, your basal metabolism should ideally be maintained at youthful levels. From the perspective of obesity, basal metabolism, as reflected in your M-Factor, can best be described as a measurement of how much fat you burn while you are sleeping.

It has often been said that the only way to really become rich is to make money while you are sleeping. **I can promise you that it is also true that the only way you can control your weight is to lose fat while you are sleepin**g. And the only way to do this is to optimize your M-Factor.

The process of optimizing your M-Factor literally involves each and every one of the "secrets" I've put forward in this book. Often the most crucial aspects are a reduction in dietary carbohydrate combined with circuit training, exercising at your FBR, adequate sleep, and natural hormone replacement. Having an optimal M-Factor forms the basis for what I refer to as permanent metabolic weight loss.

You're Not Too Fat - You're Too Weak

The more I have researched into the dynamics of what makes some people thin and others fat, the more I have begun to appreciate the importance of muscle mass. I am convinced that the lowered M-Factor consistently seen in every obese person is due to decreased muscle mass more than any other single factor.

I am so convinced of this that I tell my patients that for purposes of permanent weight control it is much more important for them to gain muscle than to lose fat. The decrease in muscle mass is the result of crash dieting, genetics, hormonal imbalances, aging, and lack of proper exercise. Careful attention to all of these factors is critical to success. Any weight loss program that doesn't seriously focus on increasing muscle mass is doomed to failure.

How To Increase Your Energy And Lose Fat Permanently

❑ Step 1 Diagnosing Insulin Resistance

Do you have insulin resistance going on in your body that is contributing to excess weight?

The most reliable way I have yet found to assess the presence and degree of insulin resistance is to analyze the C-Factor (again, see discussion of this in Chapter 3). Patients with insulin resistance will always have a C-Factor above 78. The higher the C-Factor, the more insulin resistance that is present.

Another easy, and almost as reliable method to find insulin resistance is to simply check a fasting insulin blood level. The normal range for fasting insulin in the U.S. is 5 to 25 uiu/ml, but any values greater than 7 uiu/ml means that insulin resistance is present.

This so-called "normal" range for fasting insulin levels in the United States only serves to demonstrate how common insulin resistance is, since it means that statistically speaking, more than half of the "healthy" people in the United States have significant insulin resistance.

Is it just coincidental that half the population in the U.S. is insulin resistant and half the population is obese? I don't think so. I believe it just indicates that insulin resistance is the cause of obesity in the overwhelming number of patients. Insulin levels need to be brought down below a minimum of 10 uiu/ml *before* successful fat loss can occur.

An additional sensitive way to make the diagnosis is with a fasting blood lipid test. Since insulin acts to divert foods to fat, it causes an elevation of fats in the blood. An elevation in cholesterol and triglycerides alerts me to the possibility of excess insulin. An elevation of a fraction of triglycerides known as VLDL (very low density lipoprotein) is a particularly strong indicator.

❏ Step 2 Addressing Insulin Resistance – The Glycemic Index

Dietary carbohydrate stimulates the release of insulin, so it would seem that the most immediate and effective way to reduce the tide of insulin in the body is to reduce carbohydrate consumption.

Eating carbohydrates stimulates the release of insulin in everyone. However, some people release much more insulin than normal after a carbohydrate meal. This condition is referred to as carbohydrate sensitivity, and if you have it, you should be careful not to eat more carbohydrate than you actually need.

How much should you cut back?

That varies greatly from person to person. A useful guide is to keep cutting carbohydrates back until the C-Factor is under 78, and the fasting insulin is less than 10 uiu/ml. In some cases almost all dietary carbohydrate must be eliminated in order to achieve these goals.

Researchers have discovered that certain carbohydrates stimulate the release of more insulin than others and have created a ranking of carbohydrates according to their insulin effect. This list is known as The Glycemic Index.

Here is how it works:

Carbohydrates designated with a "high glycemic" rating mean they cause the release of excess insulin. Middle and low glycemic carbohydrates release progressively less insulin.

Carbohydrate sensitive individuals should decrease the consumption of carbohydrates in general, but should particularly avoid the foods that have a high glycemic rating.

Limited amounts of low or middle glycemic carbohydrates may be permitted on an individual basis.

Note: The glycemic index does not list foods such as vegetables, meats, seeds, and dairy products because these foods have an extremely low insulin effect.

The Glycemic Index

High Glycemic Rating

1. Bread (white or whole grain, it makes no difference), pastry, cookies, crackers, pretzels, pancakes. Basically anything made from flour with the exception of pasta.

2. Rice (both white and brown), corn, millet, barley, chips, cold breakfast cereals (including muesli), cooked cereals (with the one exception of slow cooked oatmeal).

3. Bananas, pineapple, raisins, melons, mango, papaya, pumpkin.

4. All sweets. This means anything that tastes sweet, including honey, fruit juices, corn syrup, maple syrup, high fructose corn syrup, maltose, barley malt, maltodextrin, sugar, and molasses. Always check ingredient labels for sugars. Anything that ends in the suffix "ose" is a sugar. Non high glycemic sweetners are pure fructose, sucralose, xylitol and the herb stevia.

5. All root vegetables, with the exception of yams. This includes potatoes, carrots, sweet potatoes, and beets.

6. Beer and wine (even the low alcohol kind). All liquor other than vodka and gin.

Middle Glycemic

1. Oranges, peaches, plums, pears, and apples.

2. High protein pasta, yams, and "Ezekial" brand bread.

3. Peas, pinto beans, garbanzo beans, kidney beans (canned), and navy beans.

4. Vodka and Gin

Low Glycemic

1. Kidney beans, lentils, black-eyed peas, chick peas, lima beans.

2. Soy beans and soy products such as tofu, soy protein, tempeh, and miso. Be aware that soy products will often contain sugar.

3. Nuts, milk, apricots, grapes, grapefruit, cherries, berries.

4. Slow cooked oatmeal and 100% whole grain rye bread.

5. Fructose. This is the only low glycemic sugar. It is quite sweet.

❑ Step 3 Diet Concerns

Besides monitoring your intake of carbohydrates, there are three other dietary considerations that must be addressed.

The first relates to total calories. In order to lose weight, total calories must be carefully restricted. That means restricted enough to result in fat loss, but not enough to cause muscle loss.

The correct caloric intake is extremely important and very individual, and is another reason why Bio-Energy Testing™ is so helpful. Through it you can determine your basal metabolic rate. Increase this number by 20 percent and that's the number of calories you should eat per day to lose weight.

The second key consideration is to avoid hydrogenated and partially hydrogenated oils. These manmade oils are incorporated into the membranes of every cell in your body and interfere with the essential functions of the membrane. Their negative effect may well be a major contributor in the development of insulin resistance.

Hydrogenated oils are commonly found in margarine, mayonnaise, baked goods, and almost any packaged convenience food.

The third consideration is to learn to be comfortable with hunger. When you are hungry, it indicates that your glycogen stores are exhausted, and that you are meeting your energy requirements from your fat reserves. This is exactly what losing fat is all about.

If you feel hungry between meals, just relax. Remember that it's absolutely OK to be hungry. In many cases it is even necessary in order to be successful. Don't immediately run to the cookie jar or pull out a 40-30-30 bar from your desk drawer. Drink a glass of water, coffee, or tea and get on with your day. You will often find that the hunger lessens as you get over the hump, and you begin to access your fat stores better. Don't yield to hunger. Don't forget that the majority of the time we feel hunger, it is for emotional reasons.

❑ Step 4 Supplements

Nutritional deficiencies are often lurking behind insulin resistance.

Missing or deficient nutrients cannot be adequately supplied by a good diet in the case of people who are genetically susceptible to insulin resistance. Supplementation is needed. As I mentioned in the chapter on supplements, these nutrients must be taken in the correct form and dosage in order to be effective.

That's where QuickStart™ comes in. It contains all the necessary nutrients in their proper potency. This all-in-one supplement is a key element for my patients with stubborn weight problems.

One scoop of QuickStart™ is blended with one tablespoon of flax oil, with its payload of essential fatty acids. Drink it as a smoothie in the morning and afternoon.

Patients with mild insulin resistance are usually able to resolve the problem by avoiding high glycemic carbohydrates, taking the supplements that I recommend, and exercising regularly. Obese individuals require the additional help of the following supplements:

Carnitine L-carnitine is the building block for the enzyme carnitine acyltransferase, which functions in the mitochondria to facilitate the metabolism of fat. In the absence of adequate levels of l-carnitine, fat metabolism becomes seriously impaired. Since carnitine is naturally found only in meats, vegetarians are often deficient. Anthropological studies suggest that the diet of our ancient ancestors usually contained between 2-3,000 milligrams of l-carnitine, but today's diets often have less than 500 milligrams. Typical supplement dosages are from 500 to 1,000 milligrams, taken three times per day.

Coenzyme Q10 This vitamin-like substance, naturally produced in the body, is a key ingredient for cellular energy production. It becomes depleted as we age, or as a result of poor diet and taking cholesterol lowering drugs. Not surprisingly, it is often deficient in obese people. If your fasting blood coenzyme Q10 level is below 1.5 mg/l, you should supplement at a high enough dosage to reach this minimum level. Typical dosages are in the range of 30-100 milligrams per day. To enhance absorption, coenzyme Q10 should be taken with a meal which contains some fat.

Alpha Lipoic Acid This major antioxidant also becomes depleted as we age. Since alpha lipoic acid is important in the functioning of insulin receptors, a deficiency can cause insulin resistance. The recommended dose is 100-200 milligrams daily.

Conjugated Linoleic Acid (CLA) There are several studies in both humans and animals verifying the fat metabolizing effect of conjugated linoleic acid (CLA), a naturally occurring fatty acid amply contained in animal fats. Vegetarians tend to be particularly low in this oil. CLA, at doses ranging from 1000-2000 milligrams three times a day, also helps lower the insulin level.

Growth Hormone Stimulators The amino acids l-lysine and l-glutamine prompt the body to produce extra growth hormone. This is especially useful in a weight management program because obese persons are often deficient in growth hormone. You may recall from the previous chapter that growth hormone is <u>the</u> key hormone in maintaining an optimal fat to muscle ratio, so you can see how important it is for weight control.

Take 3000 milligrams of l-lysine on an empty stomach when you first wake up in the morning. Take 2000 milligrams of l-glutamine on an empty stomach at bedtime.

❑ Step 5 Natural Hormonal Replacement

The hormone deficiencies most often responsible for the low energy production causing obesity are progesterone (in women), testosterone (in women and men), the adrenal and thyroid hormones, and growth hormone.

Overcoming obesity very often requires careful replacement of these hormones on an individual basis. I suggest consulting a physician specializing in anti-aging medicine who is experienced in working with natural hormones.

A weight loss program may not succeed without such replacement.

❑ Step 6 Correct Exercise

I discussed at length the role of exercise for weight loss in my Secret No. 6. Let me quickly summarize that information here.

FBR Training When you exercise at a heart rate equal to your FBR (fat burning rate), your body is burning fat as fast as it can. As the exertion level goes beyond this point, the proportion of energy produced from fat metabolism actually decreases until you reach a point at which you don't burn fat at all. Unfortunately, due to their energy production deficit, and insulin irregularity, obese persons commonly spend all of their exercise time at this latter level. Instead of burning fat, they are only burning their limited supply of glycogen.

New patients who are obese tell me that no matter how hard they exercise they can't lose weight. No wonder. They just haven't learned the mechanics of their fat metabolism.

Proper exercise for fat loss means spending *more time* at a *lower level* of exertion. This means a minimum of forty-five to sixty minutes a day exercising at the FBR. For individuals with an aversion to exercise, this is good news indeed. Exercising at this level is very comfortable. So comfortable in fact that you could be exercising at this rate while talking on the phone, and the person you are talking to would never guess that you were exercising at all.

Exercising at your FBR, for example on a treadmill or stationary bicycle is the perfect kind of exercise to do while watching TV or reading.

Circuit Training

This is form of exercise that I generally recommend to patients. Refer to p. 106 for the details on how to do it.

Basic Pointers

Rome wasn't built in a day. Neither will you get in shape the first day, or maybe even the first month. In fact when you first start exercising you will probably not be able to do half as much as you would like to. Just be patient. It will all come around as you continue forward and get in progressively better shape.

Perform the FBR training three days a week, and the circuit training three days a week. Take one day a week off to rest and be lazy. A successful program will usually result in anywhere from 10-15 pounds the first few weeks. Most of this is water loss so don't get too excited.

After this initial period expect to lose about 1-2 pounds of weight per week. This rate of weight loss may not seem like much after hearing all the crash diet adds, but remember that with this program you are losing fat, not muscle. Ultimately this translates out to the long term success you're really looking for.

When you have lost the weight, you will only need to exercise for 30 minutes three times a week to maintain your health and optimum energy production.

❑ Step 7 Sleep, Sunlight, and Water

I can't emphasize enough the importance of adequate rest in order for your body to generate good energy. Be sure to get in seven or eight hours of quality sleep on most nights. *This often means disciplining yourself to go to bed earlier.*

And while I am in an emphasis mode, I should also remind you about getting enough sunlight and drinking enough water. Getting enough sleep, sunlight and water is free, at least so far. But even though they cost you nothing, please don't think they are any less important than the other issues I have been discussing. It may not be obvious, but sleep, sunlight, and water are all important for helping you with your weight problem, and putting you on the fast track to high energy.

The Shallenberger Blue Plate Special
(Food, Supplements, and Drinks
for a More Streamlined You)

Carefully follow the instructions below. They work! In almost all cases this approach will lead to one to two pounds of fat loss per week.

Food

Breakfast

One scoop of QuickStart™ blended with two teaspoons of flax oil.

Eggs, meats (red meat, poultry, or fish), and regular, unsweetened yogurt are optional.

Lunch

Salad with dressing, cheese, and meats, or stir-fried vegetables with meat.

3pm Snack

One scoop of QuickStart™ blended with two teaspoons of flax oil.

Supper

Meats, vegetables, salad, beans.

Snacks

A little of what you had the last meal.

Desserts

One piece of whole fresh fruit from the middle or low glycemic list after supper.

Exceptions

Two meals per week with rice, bread or soy based pasta.

General Eating Guidelines

Eat slowly and relaxed. Chew your food well. Enjoy your meals. Eat only what you need. You may have cream, salt, and spices as desired. You may use one tablespoon of fructose or xylitol a day as a sweetener. Do not eat anything for at least three hours before bedtime.

Drinks

Water is your preferred beverage. See my Secret No. 1 for how much to drink.

Definitely limit your diet sodas. One per day, if at all.

Two 4-ounce cups of coffee or green tea per day are permitted.

Herbal tea is unlimited.

No fruit juice.

Supplements (available at health food stores)

Immediately after you wake up, take 2 grams of l-lysine with a glass of water. Wait at least forty-five minutes before eating.

As noted above, take QuickStart™ in the morning and around 3 pm.

Take 2000 milligrams of conjugated linoleic acid (CLA) three times per day.

Take 100 milligrams of coenzymeQ10, 1 gram of l-carnitine, and 100 milligrams of alpha lipoic acid two times per day. You can take them with the QuickStart™.

Take 2 grams of l-glutamine at bedtime.

Laurie's Case

When I first saw Laurie she was 43-years old and weighed 220 pounds. Most of her weight gain occurred during the previous nine years, a prolonged period of marital and job stress. During this time she exercised only sporadically. She had gone on several diets, lost 20 or 30 pounds, but soon put the weight back on each time. Now, she complained, "I can't seem to lose weight no matter what I do."

Sound familiar?

Before her weight explosion years before, Laurie had weighed 150 pounds and had felt and looked great at that weight. But now, at 220, bio-impedance measurement revealed that her body fat percentage was almost 50 percent. Virtually half of her was fat! That meant 110 pounds as fat, and the other 110 pounds reflecting her lean body mass, which essentially equates to her muscle mass.

Nine years ago, before she had gained all the weight, and assuming she had a healthy body fat percentage of about 22 percent, her fat would have been 30 pounds and her muscle mass 120 pounds.

So what was her problem? Was it that she gained eighty pounds of fat, or that she lost ten pounds of muscle mass?

The answer is that the ten pounds of muscle loss is actually more of a contributing factor to her obesity than the eighty pounds of fat. This is because muscle tissue is extremely active metabolically, and burns a significant amount of fat calories even while we sleep. The more muscle mass you have, reflected by a greater lean body mass percentage, the greater will be your daily fat calorie expenditure. Laurie's ten-pound decrease in muscle mass, though it doesn't sound like much, was easily enough to prevent her from successfully burning her fat stores.

Every time Laurie embarked on a weight loss plan, she lost much more than she bargained for. Each time she had indeed lost weight. But the lost weight included muscle loss, because weight loss plans do not focus on the real problem with obesity, a decreased M-Factor. In fact, weight loss programs only aggravate the situation because calorie restriction causes the body to lower its M-Factor even more.

The only way to lose just fat without any muscle loss is by taking measures to increase your M-Factor. Bio-Energy Testing™ is invaluable not only to help you know how to do that, but also to insure that your effort is in fact actually raising the M-Factor.

Laurie's muscle loss also amplified another problem. It increased her insulin resistance. This is because muscle cells have an enormous amount of insulin receptors. Loss of muscle mass therefore results in a loss of total body insulin receptors, causing an elevated insulin level.

Because her muscle loss caused her M-Factor to decrease and her insulin resistance to increase, Laurie ultimately regained back all the fat she had lost...and then some. *She gained back the fat, but unfortunately not the muscle.* This "yo-yo" effect over the years, in combination with incorrect exercising habits, caused her to lose enough muscle to put her in a hole she couldn't escape from.

But it wasn't just a lack of exercise and repeated dieting that caused her problems. It was also the fact that she had gone from being a 34-year-old woman to a 43-year-old, and had now developed the hormonal deficiencies that come with aging. One of the most common effects associated with these deficiencies is a loss of muscle mass. All these elements fit into the equation of solving Laurie's weight problem.

Laurie's Case Resolved:

Hormonal Replacement and Correct Exercise

The first thing we did was to put Laurie through Bio-Energy Testing™. The results provided the necessary information to customize a personal and effective program for this unhappy woman.

The data indicated that low thyroid activity was significantly depressing her M-Factor. Not surprisingly, all her previous thyroid blood tests were within the normal range. I prescribed thyroid replacement to increase her M-Factor to normal.

Bio-Energy Testing™ also determined her FBR and ATR. I explained to Laurie that she needed to begin exercising three days per week, for 45 to 60 minutes at her FBR. Another three days per week she was to do circuit training. She was scheduled with our clinic trainer to learn how to do this, and every 6-8 weeks she would again meet with the trainer to update her progress, and alter her exercise protocol as needed.

Next, Bio-Energy Testing™ revealed a C-Factor of 93. You may recall from my discussion in Chapter 3 that this is a key measurement of fat metabolism and carbohydrate intake. Her result clearly indicated she was consuming far too many carbohydrates. I did not restrict her total calories because she was not overeating but I recommended she drastically limit her carbohydrates.

Finally, hormone testing revealed she was in a state of relative estrogen excess, and that she was depleted of DHEA. As an anabolic hormone DHEA is very much involved in the production of muscle tissue. I was not surprised she was low in DHEA. DHEA is also extremely valuable in correcting insulin resistance.

To correct these imbalances, I prescribed a DHEA supplement and a topical progesterone cream to balance out her estrogen. All hormone levels were regularly rechecked to ensure that she was being administered the correct doses for her individual needs. An additional benefit of QuickStart™ is that it stimulates the liver to lower elevated estrogen levels.

Laurie was determined to beat her weight problem. So, armed with new information and several natural prescriptions, she set off to remake herself. And she did great. Within a year she had lost 55 pounds of fat. More importantly, she had gained 5 pounds of muscle through her exercise program.

Now, more than three years later, she has her former figure back, and continues to maintain her desired weight simply by following the guidelines I have outlined in the book.

As an additional reward for her tenacity, Laurie no longer needed to adhere so strictly to carbohydrate avoidance, because her fat loss, muscle gain, and hormonal replacement had completely eliminated her insulin resistance. She had literally made her body over.

Laurie's case is not exceptional. In fact, it is rather typical. When energy production is normalized it is possible for any obese individual to achieve - and maintain - a permanent and healthy weight level.

My Recommendations:

❑ Carefully follow the food and supplement instructions above.

❑ Obtain a weight composition analysis through bio-impedance testing, available at most health spas. The ideal body fat percentages are 18 to 22 percent for women and 12 to 18 percent for men. If your measurements are in line, follow my recommendations to avoid developing a weight problem as you age.

❑ If your body fat percentage is above these levels, you have a weight problem that needs to be resolved. The most efficient way to do that is to obtain Bio-Energy Testing™. See Chapter 3 for the details. The test will provide you with your particular exercise zones, and accurately measure your M-Factor and your C-Factor.

❑ Regardless of what thyroid blood tests show, if your M-Factor is below normal, you may very likely need thyroid hormone replacement to be successful. You must take enough thyroid to bring your M-Factor into the optimal range of 90-100. If your physician isn't familiar with physiological hormonal replacement and won't prescribe thyroid replacement unless the blood tests are out of the normal range, I suggest finding a doctor who can help you. For a referral, contact either the American College for the Advancement of Medicine (949-583-7666, or www.acam.org on the Internet), or the American Academy of Anti-Aging Medicine (719-475-8775, or www.worldhealth.net).

❑ Exercise three days a week for 45-60 minutes at your FBR. Spend another three days with 35-40 minutes of circuit training.

❑ Obtain another Bio-Energy Testing™ analysis after every 25-30 pounds of fat loss. The reason for this is that energy measurements will improve as weight comes off. The program will have to be adjusted accordingly.

❑ As you lose weight you can also monitor progress from time-to-time with additional bio-impedance analysis. Remember, a correct exercise program will result in putting on muscle weight even as you lose fat weight. So your overall weight may not reflect your net fat loss. The best way to follow your results is by bio-impedance analysis. You can also measure your waist, thighs, and hips, and take a good look in the mirror as you take off the weight and tone yourself up.

❑ The hormones intimately involved with weight management are the thyroid hormones, estrogen, progesterone, testosterone, DHEA, and growth hormone. Unless your physician has been trained in natural hormone replacement, you will need a specialist in this field. Contact the organizations listed above for a referral.

❑ On a routine basis, practice breath meditation, drink plenty of water, get plenty of sunlight, and have a full night of sleep.

Secret No. 10
Disease Prevention

The recommendations you've been reading throughout the book can take you far along the path of anti-aging and preventing the diseases of aging. In this chapter I would like to address issues related to the prevention and treatment of several common conditions: cardiovascular disorders, cancer, osteoporosis, and diabetes.

Cardiovascular Disorders

(Atherosclerosis, Strokes, And Heart Disease)

Vascular disease, also known as arteriosclerosis, develops when blood vessels become hard, stiff, and inflexible. If this occurs in the major arteries leading to the heart or the brain the consequences can be serious and life threatening.

The most common type of this disease is atherosclerosis, a term adopted from the Greek words athero (meaning gruel or paste) and sclerosis (hardness).

The Greeks had it right. In this condition, plaque deposits form on the inner lining of the arteries. They are made from fat, mostly cholesterol, and then become hardened by the deposition of calcium.

The result is a hardening and narrowing of the arteries and reduction of vital blood flow. This reduction in circulation deprives cells throughout the body of oxygen and essential nutrients. When this process becomes advanced in arteries leading to the heart, you can develop chest pain (angina) and heart attacks, the No. 1 disease killer. When it involves arteries leading to the brain, or in small arteries within the brain, you can develop stroke or senility.

Atherosclerosis is also a major contributor to premature aging because the decrease in circulation means less oxygen and nutrients reaching the cells for energy production.

Scientific evidence indicates that atherosclerosis is completely preventable. **When I say completely, I mean 100 percent.**

With what we currently know today, this condition and all the diseases and suffering associated with it, can be completely eradicated. But to understand how to eliminate this problem, you must first have an understanding of what causes it.

What Causes Atherosclerosis?

Most people, when asked, would simply pin the blame on too much cholesterol in the blood resulting from too much cholesterol in the diet.

This answer contains but a small shred of the truth. *Cholesterol is only one of many different factors, and is, in fact, a relatively minor one at that.* It is not the Great Satan of Heart Disease as we have been led to believe. And I will talk more about that misconception in a moment.

The beginnings of atherosclerosis occur with damage to the inner lining of the artery. The primary factors involved in this initiating injury are well known, and happily, all of them are treatable. Let's examine each of them here:

❏ Exaggerated Stress Response

Hardening of the arteries seem to be accompanied by a hardening of attitude. As people get older, they tend to react more to stress than when they were younger. This results from an accumulation of attitudes such as inflexibility, clinging on to grief, guilt, regrets, and resentment from old hurts, a lost sense of purpose, decreased appreciation of beauty, and fear of death and disease. Over the years this kind of stress causes adrenaline-induced free radical damage, increased cholesterol levels, and high blood pressure, all of which damage arteries.

There are many cures for dealing with stress. Breath meditation. Exercise. Rest. Spending quality time with grandkids or friends. Pursuing a hobby that unleashes unexpressed creativity within us. Good companionship. A pet.

The key is finding things in life, no matter how old we are or what misfortunes have befallen us, that bring us joy and nourish the heart and mind. This is what dissolves stress.

Inevitably, the two components that are the most crucial to successfully dealing with all the stresses that come with modern day living are a *daily routine* that includes adequate time for these healthful activities, and the *personal discipline* needed to adhere to it.

You are probably aware of the amazing studies published over the years by Dean Ornish, M.D. Ornish has clearly demonstrated that coronary artery disease can often be reversed simply by stress management techniques such as meditation and yoga, along with proper diet and exercise.

❑ Hormonal Deficiencies

The most significant deficiencies leading to atherosclerosis involve estrogen, testosterone, thyroid, growth hormone, and DHEA. Natural hormone replacement is one of the most effective ways to keep your arteries soft and pliable (see my Secret No. 8).

❑ Mineral Deficiencies

A proper diet, as I defined earlier (Secret No. 4), minimizes the risk of mineral deficiency. However, due to commercial farming methods, the use of synthetic fertilizers, and the processing of food, our meals are often short of key minerals that contribute to healthy arteries. The most common deficiencies I find among my patients are zinc, chromium, and magnesium. The literature is replete with studies connecting deficiencies of critical minerals to atherosclerosis.

In one 1984 study entitled, "Low plasma chromium in patients with coronary artery and heart diseases," which appeared in *Biological Trace Element Research*, every patient with arteriographic evidence of coronary artery disease was found to have a low chromium level. By comparison, only 20 percent of patients without disease had a low level. Laboratory experiments have shown as much as a 50 percent reduction in atherosclerotic plaques when animals are supplemented with chromium.

According to a study entitled "Magnesium and trace minerals: risk factors for coronary heart disease," published in the prestigious cardiovascular journal *Circulation*, magnesium deficiency is associated with an increased risk of coronary artery disease, sudden cardiac death, myocardial infarction, and fatal arrhythmias.

Using a new technology known as electron beam coronary tomography, researchers have been able to document that coronary artery disease is directly correlated with increased levels of calcium in the coronary arteries. Magnesium supplementation decreases the calcium content of these arteries, making them much less likely to develop atherosclerosis.

Regular supplementation that includes these minerals is critical, even if you are eating a perfect diet.

❑ Chronic Heavy Metal Poisoning

Toxic metals present in our air, water, and food build up in our bodies over decades. In particular, lead, arsenic, and cadmium contribute to arterial damage. The most common source is drinking water. Yet another reason to drink only filtered water.

Once inside, your body cannot readily excrete them. They become deposited in the tissues, particularly the arteries, and accumulate over the years.

This is graphically demonstrated by provocative testing, a technique offered by many practitioners of alternative medicine. The method involves the administration of chelating drugs, substances that have the ability to bind to heavy metals stuck in the arteries and other tissues and promote their excretion through the urine.

By obtaining a urine specimen before and after the chelating drug is administered we are able to discover the full extent of the heavy metal poisoning that is present. It is quite common, in fact it is the rule, that the pre-provocative urine specimen will show very little or no heavy metals while the post-provocative specimen will be loaded. This demonstrates two principles of heavy metals. One, simply examining the blood or urine for heavy metals without using a provocative chelating drug is often useless in documenting their presence. Two, without the use of chelating drugs, they won't be removed.

Chronic heavy metal poisoning is a common cause of an abnormally low E.Q.

❏ Inadequate Sleep

Lack of adequate sleep is a documented cause of diabetes, hypertension, and obesity, all of which are contributors to atherosclerosis. See my Secret No. 2.

❏ Poor Cardiovascular Conditioning

This means not enough exercise, and specifically, not enough of the right amount and right kind of exercise. See my Secret No. 6.

Bio-Energy Testing™ routinely discovers the inability of the typical over-50 heart at providing adequate oxygen to the cells and tissues. Among the cells that suffer from this shortfall are the intimal cells that line the arterial walls. They require a high infusion of oxygen to properly function, and without adequate oxygen they become especially vulnerable to the processes that cause atherosclerosis. Regular exercise can prevent and even reverse poor cardiovascular functioning, provide an increased supply of oxygen to the intimal cells, and reduce atherosclerosis.

❏ Obesity and Insulin Resistance

These conditions are almost always found together. See my Secret No. 9 on how to test for and treat these problems.

❑ Elevated Homocysteine Level

Homocysteine is a naturally occurring amino acid in the body. Under normal circumstances it is rapidly cleared by the liver with the help of vitamins B-6, folic acid, B-12, and food substances known as methyl donors. But deficiencies of these vitamins and/or sub-optimal liver function commonly result in an elevated homocysteine level. That spells trouble.

The excess homocysteine triggers harmful reactions that initiate damage in the arterial walls. Studies confirm that about 10 percent of all deaths from atherosclerosis occur as a result of an elevated homocysteine level.

Patients with a family history of heart attacks below the age of sixty are considered at risk for developing elevated homocysteine.

Supplementation with the key vitamins, and maintaining a healthy liver, can prevent a homocysteine buildup.

Excessive homocysteine, by the way, has effects beyond the arteries. According to a recent study in the *Annals of the New York Academy of Sciences*, it can also cause chromosomal damage. Such damage is a major sign of aging.

Other studies have shown that people with even a moderate elevation have as much as a 50 percent increased risk of dying from all causes of illness when compared to individuals with a low level of homocysteine. Elevated levels have also been recently implicated as a cause of Alzheimer's.

Laboratory reports describe the average range of homocysteine to be between 5 and 15 umol/l, but optimal levels are below 7 umol/l.

❑ Lipoprotein (a)

Elevated blood lipoprotein (a) has received less attention than homocysteine, and certainly much, much less than cholesterol, but it is arguably the single most significant risk factor for heart disease.

Like cholesterol, another type of lipoprotein, this substance is an extremely sticky molecule. As it circulates in the blood it has a marked tendency to adhere to sites of arterial wall damage and contribute to plaque buildup, atherosclerosis, and arterial blockades. This tendency is greater than any other lipid.

Lipoprotein (a) also exerts a negative effect on the clotting mechanisms of blood, and thus creates an additional risk factor for heart attacks and stroke. The "acceptable" range for lipo (a) is up to 80 mg/dl (some laboratories have an acceptable ceiling as high as 130 mg/dl!), but the optimal level is below 20 mg/dl.

Linus Pauling, one of the greatest scientific geniuses of the 20th century, argued almost thirty years ago that an elevated lipoprotein (a) level was perhaps the leading risk factor for heart disease.

You haven't heard more about this substance for a simple reason. Pharmaceutical companies have not yet been able to patent a drug to lower it. When they do, you can expect a high decibel campaign about a completely new discovery. This is a sad commentary on the way medicine is practiced in this country. Instead of being driven by physicians and patients, those who care the most, the system is driven by pharmaceutical corporations with an overriding interest in the bottom line.

Fortunately, we don't have to wait for the drug industry. We already have a solution. It is not patentable, but it works. Years ago Pauling demonstrated that deficiencies of lysine (a naturally occurring amino acid) and vitamin C were the main causes of elevated lipoprotein (a). With the additional support of B vitamins, a low carbohydrate diet, and hormone replacement therapy, this dangerous sticky stuff can be kept in its place.

❑ Coenzyme Q10 Deficiency

CoQ10 is a vitamin-like substance and a fundamental ingredient in the cellular conversion of oxygen to energy. Therefore, any decrease threatens your energy production and promotes the possibility of many related problems. Depletion is associated with aging, poor diet, the use of cholesterol-lowering drugs, diabetes and heart disease.

Adequate CoQ10 is necessary for the integrity of all tissues, and even more so for those tissues with a high metabolic need for energy such as the heart, liver, and brain. Studies show that patients with heart disease are deficient in CoQ10. And deficiencies can also lead to high blood pressure, according to Texas cardiologist Peter Langsjoen, M.D., who has been using CoQ10 in his practice for nearly twenty years. Chronic high blood pressure causes the arteries to become constricted, and choke off the blood supply to the heart.

For reasons not yet fully understood, CoQ10 levels often becomes depleted as we age. Although CoQ10 is made in every cell in the body, the CoQ10 found circulating in the blood comes primarily from the liver. **The liver synthesizes it from the lower forms of the enzyme such as CoQ6 and CoQ8 which are found in vegetables.** Yet another reason your liver is the most important organ in your body. The laboratory reports the statistical range for serum CoQ10 to be between .75 and 1.5, but most research indicates that levels above 1.5 are required for optimal health.

Experts strongly recommend supplementation with CoQ10 to remedy a possible deficiency, and particularly for people in middle age and above.

For sure, anyone taking a cholesterol drug should be on a CoQ10 supplement. Failure to do so means substituting one relatively minor risk factor (high cholesterol) for a much more significant one (CoQ10 deficiency).

❏ Elevated Iron

The iron story is fascinating. Women, as is well known, have a much lower incidence of heart disease than men and also live an average of 10 to 15 percent longer. This difference exists in every culture studied, regardless of diet, exercise, and stress, with one exception: men who regularly donate blood. They basically share the same desirable statistics as women.

The explanation for these interesting observations most likely has to do with iron. Inside the body, iron is a two-edged sword. On the one hand it is of paramount importance to the production of energy. It is iron that chemically binds to oxygen in hemoglobin molecules in the blood and carries it for delivery to the cells. But it is also iron, in excess, that instigates damaging free radical activity. Damage from free radicals is a major factor in the degenerative processes of aging and diseases such as atherosclerosis.

Menstruating women obviously have less iron because of their cyclic blood loss. But many men, due to their inherited genetics and the effects of the male hormone testosterone, have a tendency to develop a higher iron level. This condition is also found in some post-menopausal women.

Excessive dietary consumption of iron from supplements or due to the use of iron cookware can also be a contributing factor. The potential for iron overload is why I have never added iron to QuickStart™.

An excessive iron level can be discovered by examining the blood ferritin level. Ferritin is an iron binding protein that stores iron in the liver. A blood test revealing an elevated ferritin level often indicates an excess of iron in the body.

I routinely check the ferritin level of patients and find that 10 to 15 percent of men and 3 to 5 percent of post menopausal women have an elevated level. For such patients, I make sure they carefully avoid iron supplements. I also recommend they regularly donate blood. In addition, there are natural substances such as colostrum, garlic, and algae that are able to reduce iron.

The statistical range for serum ferritin in most laboratories is usually between 40-180 ng/ml, but I believe, as do many experts, that any value over 70 ng/ml can indicate an excessive tissue iron burden.

❑ Antioxidant Deficiencies

Free radicals are highly reactive molecular fragments formed in the course of every day energy production in the cells. In excess they cause considerable damage to cells and tissues, and thus participate in disease processes and accelerated aging.

The body has evolved an elaborate defense system of enzymes and other substances called antioxidants to prevent such a destructive excess. This system is stimulated by acrobic exercise and weakened by stress and infection. The system is also undermined by exposure to drugs, pesticides, and other chemicals.

Free radicals are always involved in the initial arterial damage leading to atherosclerotic plaques.

Certain nutrients are required to keep the antioxidant system running strong. Among them are vitamins, minerals, and amino acids. Fortunately, you can purchase these substances in health food stores and drug stores. Chief among them are vitamins C and E, CoQ10, alpha lipoic acid, the amino acid cysteine, and the minerals zinc, copper, manganese, and selenium.

These supplements can help your body's fight against free radicals and also help prevent the development of atherosclerosis.

❑ Elevated Triglycerides

Triglycerides are fats that circulate in the blood. They are produced in the body from carbohydrates. An elevated level suggests an increased risk for cardiovascular disease (as well as breast cancer), and is also indicative of eating a diet too high in carbohydrates. High triglycerides tend to be ignored by many physicians because there is no patentable drug to treat it.

The influence of triglycerides on atherosclerosis seems in large part related to HDL, the so-called "good" cholesterol. High triglycerides cause a decrease in HDL.

Harvard researcher Michael Gaziano, M.D., pointed out the significance of this relationship in a 1997 article in the cardiology journal *Circulation*. He found that individuals with the highest ratio (high triglycerides and low HDL) were sixteen times more likely to have a heart attack than those with the lowest ratio.

Ideally, triglyceride levels should be below 120 mg/dl. An ideal HDL/ triglyceride ratio is one to two, and anything over one to three should be treated.

Improving the ratio can be readily achieved through weight loss, exercise, a low carbohydrate diet, and supplementation with fish oils, l-carnitine, and niacin.

❏ **Hypertension**

The relationship between hypertension and atherosclerosis is well known. Simply put, elevated pressure in the arteries is a significant cause of atherosclerosis.

More than 50 million Americans have this condition, also called high blood pressure.

The standard treatment is anti-hypertensive medication. However, as strange as it may seem, many of the medications used to treat high blood pressure actually promote atherosclerosis. This is particularly true of medications known as diuretics and beta-blockers.

In most cases hypertension responds quite well to a combination of treatments focusing on weight loss, exercise, a low carbohydrate diet, heavy metal chelation, and supplementation with CoQ10.

Breath meditation (see my Secret No. 7) is also beneficial because it helps relieve stress, a major contributor to hypertension.

Stress is often related to time urgency, the feeling that there just isn't enough time to accomplish what needs to be done. It will always be more attractive for the time-urgent individual to take a blood pressure pill in three seconds than to alter the diet, meditate, exercise, and take supplements, but for those who really want to live longer and better, the correct choice is clear.

For patients with severe hypertension and who have been on medication for many years it may be difficult to eliminate the drugs. But often the alternative approach allows a reduction in medication dosage.

Your blood pressure should ideally be at or below 120/80.

The Great Cholesterol (Mis)Conception

Cholesterol is obviously involved in atherosclerosis, but not to the degree you have been led to believe. The whole issue of cholesterol has been overblown and oversold. It has been so totally distorted that many view it as the number one public health menace.

It has become a fixation of the medical establishment and has spawned a huge industry. You have low cholesterol foods. No cholesterol foods.

Cholesterol blood tests. And, most troubling of all, the increasing promotion of a very dangerous class of pharmaceutical drugs called statins, to lower cholesterol levels. The ads are everywhere. On TV. On the radio. In newspapers and magazines. The drugs are even being promoted to healthy people as a smart prevention strategy.

As a strategy for what? In my opinion the strategy is simply one designed to make pharmaceutical companies richer.

For most people, there are many good reasons why fixating on cholesterol, and worse, trying to lower cholesterol with pharmaceutical drugs, is a dangerous and medically unsound way to prevent heart disease:

Reason No. 1

Cholesterol is only one of many factors leading to heart disease. If all risk factors aren't individually identified and treated, simply lowering cholesterol will not appreciably reduce your overall risk.

Studies *repeatedly* show that these medications demonstrate no beneficial effect at all for 70 percent of those who use them. The other 30 percent show a modest benefit at best!

Virtually all of the studies examining the effect of lowering cholesterol on the overall incidence of heart disease have been quite disappointing. One of the first and largest of such studies, the Helsinki and Oslo Heart Study, quite clearly pointed out that there is practically no reduction in death from heart attacks from the use of cholesterol lowering medication. Those on medication had a *slightly* reduced risk of heart attack, but there was *no difference* in deaths from all causes between medicated and non-medicated patients.

Reason No. 2

It is not actually cholesterol per se that damages the arteries. *It is oxidized cholesterol.* Cholesterol becomes oxidized when the body's antioxidant defenses become depleted. This occurs as a result of excess stress, inadequate fitness, and deficient intake of antioxidant nutrients. And, as I will explain in a moment, cholesterol drugs can actually suppress a major component in your protective antioxidant defenses.

Following the ten steps in this book can help prevent cholesterol from becoming oxidized and harming your arteries - no matter how elevated your cholesterol levels are.

Reason No. 3

Cholesterol medications inhibit the same enzyme system that produces coenzyme Q10, a vital compound that has indispensably essential roles in the body. CoQ10 serves as a raw material in the cellular production of energy and is a powerful antioxidant.

CoQ10 acts as a "bodyguard" for LDL cholesterol, accompanying the LDL in the bloodstream and protecting it from free radical oxidation. Recent research has found that the most susceptible LDL (LDL3) is "equipped" with CoQ10.

Research has also found that cholesterol-lowering drugs deplete the CoQ10 that your body produces. The long-term effects are potentially disastrous, and motivated the International CoQ10 Association, a group of researchers and clinicians who study the uses of CoQ10, to voice their concerns to the U.S. Food and Drug Administration. In 2001, these medical professionals urged that the FDA warn patients taking statin drugs about the CoQ10 connection. The group recommended that such patients take CoQ10 supplements to hopefully avoid a deficiency while taking these drugs.

Among other things, studies have shown that heart failure is associated with a CoQ10 deficiency. Heart cells require a huge amount of energy, and therefore, are the primary cellular consumers of CoQ10 in the body.

Why are we having a resurgence of heart failure in the U.S.? Could it be because of the effects of cholesterol medications?

CoQ10 experts tell us that people taking these drugs do not develop symptoms of possible CoQ10 deficiency immediately. After a year or two, they say, patients may complain of malaise and muscular aches and pains. It is interesting to note that recent medical reports have emerged about side effects of statins, and particularly the potential for muscle damage. One major drug was pulled off the market by the FDA in the summer of 2001!

Nobody has specifically connected the dots yet, but this could be related to CoQ10 deficiency. Muscles need energy to work, and without enough CoQ10, energy production is impaired.

Not just muscles, but all cells need CoQ10. Thus, a deficiency can have widespread medical implications. For more information on the CoQ10-statin connection, and for a medical update on this very important substance, you may want to get a copy of *The User's Guide to CoQ10* by Martin Zucker, available in most health food stores.

Common complications of statins also include paralysis and rheumatic joint disease. A report in the British medical journal *Lancet* pointed out that there is *no* overall death rate decrease from the use of cholesterol lowering drugs. That's because any reduction in cardiac deaths is offset by an increase in non-cardiac deaths.

Reason No. 4

Cholesterol lowering drugs may cause cancer. There have been several very disturbing studies on this subject that the drug companies fail to mention in their T.V. ads.

In one review article from the University of California School of Medicine entitled "Carcinogenicity of lipid-lowering drugs," the authors state the following: "All members of the two most popular classes of lipid-lowering drugs (the fibrates and the statins) cause cancer in rodents, in some cases at levels of animal exposure close to those prescribed to humans."

They go on further to state: "Longer-term clinical trials and careful postmarketing surveillance during the next several decades are needed to determine whether cholesterol-lowering drugs cause cancer in humans." Other studies on the use of these drugs have demonstrated a higher incidence of cancer in the subjects on the medications than the controls. In the meantime many physicians having been convinced by the pharmaceutical industry that these medications are helpful, are possibly placing their patients at risk for cancer.

Reason No. 5

Cholesterol is in your body for a reason.

Did you know that less than 20 percent of the cholesterol in your body comes from your diet? Most of it is made in the liver.

Apparently it is too important a molecule to be trusted to dietary intake alone.

All your steroid hormones are made from cholesterol. All your cell membranes are made from cholesterol. Your brain and nervous system are almost entirely made of cholesterol.

A low cholesterol level is associated with immune deficiency and with an increased risk of death from all causes, including cancer.

Reason No. 6

Instead of introducing a harmful medication into the system, why don't physicians correct the problem(s) that cause high cholesterol in the first place? Drugs, obviously, don't correct the causes. They just squelch the body's production of cholesterol.

Common causes of high cholesterol include low thyroid, stress, antioxidant deficiency, obesity, low DHEA, low sex hormones, insulin resistance, nutritional deficiencies, sleep deprivation, and low fiber diets.

If you have elevated cholesterol, you may have any or all of these problems. It makes more sense to correct the problems than treat the symptoms, especially in the case of elevated cholesterol. Artificially lowering cholesterol is risky business. I believe the medical profession should focus on more productive things. **In the end, perhaps the only ones really benefiting from cholesterol lowering drugs are the drug manufacturers**.

So What Really Causes Heart Attacks?

I've explained the factors that cause the constriction, hardening, and narrowing of the arteries. A significant amount of blockage in the coronary arteries supplying the heart sets up the conditions for a myocardial infarction, that is, a heart attack. But it turns out that there are often other factors that are more responsible for the actual heart attack than the blocked arteries.

Increased Clotting Tendency. The blood of many persons with coronary artery disease has a tendency to form clots at alarmingly high rates. This increased tendency causes extensive clots at plaque sites.

The situation becomes potentially deadly when a plaque becomes eroded, exposing its contents to the blood stream. The clotting elements in the blood then adhere to this vulnerable plaque which further blocks the flow of blood. Clots, or a portion of the plaque, may break off, be swept away by the blood, and contribute to a life-threatening obstruction at another damaged or narrow blood vessel juncture.

If enough blood is choked off from reaching the heart muscle the result is a heart attack.

This clotting risk can be neatly reduced by taking all of the ingredients in QuickStart™. The formula contains herbs and nutrients that effectively keep the blood thin. Often, this is the only remedy needed by my at-risk patients to correct this problem.

Infected Plaques. One rather surprising cause of heart attacks involves the immune system. Researchers have discovered that common bacteria can grow on arterial plaques. As a result of these infections, the plaques may break off and embolize further down line into the coronary artery, causing a sudden heart attack.

The discovery was made when researchers found that coronary artery disease patients regularly treated with antibiotics for other conditions were less likely to have a heart attack. Apparently patients who develop these infected plaques are unable to mount an effective immune response. The immune enhancing nutrients found in QuickStart™ along with natural hormone replacement and stress reduction, can help your immune system prevent and even eradicate such infections.

Coronary Artery Vasospasm. Vasospasm is another common prelude to chest pain and sudden cardiac arrest. The term refers to a spasm of the smooth muscles surrounding the coronary artery. The result is a tightening of the artery diameter and a decrease of the blood flow. One autopsy study indicated that up to 70 percent of heart attack deaths are preceded by a coronary artery vasospasm.

Among its many important contributions to the body, the mineral magnesium helps keep arteries nice and relaxed. Coronary artery vasospasm is almost always caused by magnesium deficiency, a frequent result of processed food diets, prolonged use of diuretics, and excessive consumption of coffee, tea, and soda pop. Magnesium supplementation (QuickStart™ is high in magnesium) can reduce the risk of vasospasm.

Poor Fat Utilization. An overlooked - and *extremely* important - element in heart attack causation relates to the poor ability of patients with coronary artery disease to optimally metabolize fat for energy. **The heart, like all the other muscles in the body, prefers to burn fat as its primary energy source**. Fat metabolism defects can be diagnosed by an elevated C-Factor and a low Fat-Power Factor. Individuals with defective fat metabolism are at a significantly increased risk for the development of a heart attack simply because their heart tissues are less metabolically active. This explains to a large extent the elevated risk for persons who are overweight and/or have a high level of fat in the blood.

The Real Facts On Bypass And Angioplasty

One of my genuine concerns is the escalating rise of various surgical plaque removal procedures such as bypass surgery and angioplasty to treat coronary artery disease. This is worrisome because these procedures entail a significant risk of death and neurological impairment, combined with a high degree of failure within five years.

Furthermore, and most importantly, they do nothing to address the causes of heart disease which I've covered here. Lastly, there are safer, more effective alternatives to these procedures that are readily available.

Clinical studies show no significant difference in survival rates between those who opt for angioplasty or bypass surgery and those who choose to treat their disease medically. Several years ago, the *New England Journal of Medicine* showcased a study demonstrating the ineffectiveness of both invasive methods to extend life following a heart attack.

In the study, researchers at the University of Toronto compared the death rate for 444 Canadian heart patients to a matched group of Americans. At the end of one year following the first heart attack, the death rate was 34 percent in both groups.

However, the crucial difference was this: 12 percent of U.S. patients underwent angioplasty, compared to 1.5 percent of the Canadians; 11.7 percent of the Americans had bypass surgery, compared again to 1.5 percent of the Canadians.

Does this study and others like it suggest there is absolutely no place for these procedures in the medical care of patients with coronary artery disease? Not at all.

But the results strongly indicate that as much as 80% of the angioplasties and bypasses performed in the United States are ineffective and unnecessary. This is a particular embarrassment, because as I mentioned above, these procedures carry a substantial risk of death and morbidity.

What's angioplasty...What's a bypass?

Coronary balloon angioplasty is an invasive method of opening blocked arteries that might impede flow to the heart and possibly result in heart attack or death. The technique involves inserting and inflating a tiny balloon into the affected blood vessel, which compresses some of the blocking plaque against the arterial wall, thus improving blood flow.

Almost one million angioplasties were performed in the United States in 1998.

In bypass surgery, the surgeon reroutes blood around clogged coronary arteries to improve the supply of blood and oxygen to the heart. This is accomplished by taking a blood vessel from another part of the body and grafting it above and below the blocked part of the affected coronary artery.

More than half-a-million bypass surgeries are performed in the U.S. each year.

Angiography Can Lead To Errors

Other studies, also published in leading journals, have demonstrated a major problem with angiographies, the main guiding diagnostic procedure used to determine whether or not a bypass or angioplasty should be performed. The findings conclude that these tests are subject to erroneous interpretation in as much as 70 percent of cases.

Adding up these studies, one reaches the rather shocking conclusion that when a physician in the United States tells a patient that an angiogram indicates the need for bypass surgery or angioplasty, there is perhaps a 70 percent chance that the interpretation is wrong. Moreover, even if the interpretation is correct, the odds are only 10-20 percent that the bypass procedure or angioplasty will actually extend life.

How can this be? It seems so natural to conclude that if you remove the blockages you eliminate the problem. But as with many things in medicine, what seems rather obvious at first glance only turns out to be a small part of the whole picture.

Angioplasty and bypass are of limited value because they don't treat the causes, that is, the factors I have cited here. They merely treat the effect. Thus the causes are still at work and the disease process still advancing.

The most effective approach to the treatment and prevention of coronary artery disease can only occur when *all* the causal factors are addressed.

In my opinion, the best therapeutic approach combines the timely and judicious application of pharmaceutical and homeopathic remedies, along with attention to all of the points I have been making.

The Value Of Chelation Therapy

I regard chelation therapy as a very safe and effective form of treatment for coronary artery disease. This method involves a series of intravenous drips using a solution of minerals, vitamins, and a special amino acid called EDTA (ethylene diamine tetracetic acid).

EDTA is an amino acid similar to those forming protein foods. It has a strong attraction for toxic metals (such as lead, cadmium, nickel, and arsenic) which it binds up and escorts out of the body. It also has the ability to bind up and remove calcium deposits that are hardening arterial plaques. As a result, arterial walls become softer with greater elasticity. This increases circulation, meaning more oxygen and nutrients get to the heart and all other cells throughout the body.

Chelation improves the function of individual cells and their enzyme systems, particularly the endothelial cells that line the arteries.

The method also infuses the body with beneficial minerals, such as potassium and magnesium, which are typically deficient in patients.

The grand effect is to significantly defuse the many risk factors that lead to heart attacks and strokes.

I offer chelation therapy to my patients in the context of a broad-based health care approach including the many steps outlined in this book. Chelation can be used along with other treatments for heart disease, such as diuretics, blood thinners, and blood pressure medication. However, I find that the need for medication is usually reduced, and sometimes even eliminated, during and following successful chelation therapy. High blood pressure is often reduced or normalized.

Chelation therapy is effective, entirely safe, and completely free of any significant side effects. Moreover, it is inexpensive. An added bonus is that it improves circulation throughout the body, not just to the heart.

For those who would like to learn more about chelation therapy, not only in coronary artery disease but in other diseases as well, there are several excellent books on the subject that can be found in the health section of any major bookstore.

To find a doctor trained in chelation therapy, contact The American College for the Advancement of Medicine at 949-583-7666 or visit the organization's web site at www.acam.org.

Unfortunately, the method is ignored or rejected by a majority of cardiologists.

I personally know a number of cardiologists who are totally convinced that chelation therapy is not nearly as effective as angioplasty or bypass surgery. When they see my patients who tell them how much chelation has helped, these doctors dismiss the improvement as a "placebo effect."

However, I should point out that I have never met a single cardiologist who called the method ineffective after giving it a decent chance. On the contrary, cardiologists I know who have been open to chelation, and witnessed the results, have never gone back to the knee jerk mentality of surgery for each and every case of advanced arterial disease.

Scare tactics usually work pretty well. I can't tell you how many times a patient of mine has been told by a well-meaning cardiologist that an "emergency" procedure is needed to "save your life," only to be successfully treated in our clinic without the need for any dangerous procedure or therapy.

Studies have shown that 89 percent of all cases of coronary artery occlusion respond well to a combination of chelation therapy and medication.

In actuality the only known "emergency" indication for surgical intervention is "uncontrolled angina."

Cancer

Strictly speaking, cancer is not a disease of aging. It can strike at any age. However, the incidence of cancer rises sharply with age, and so it is reasonable to wonder what it is about the aging process that so greatly contributes to this problem.

The starting - and startling - point to begin considering the issue is this: If you are over fifty it is very likely that you already have cancer in your body. In fact, it's almost 100 percent likely!

Autopsy studies based on individuals who died in accidents or from causes other than cancer have confirmed that nearly every person older than fifty already has at least one cancerous tumor in the body.   I am not talking about a few cancerous cells.   I mean actual cancers. And many persons, according to these studies, were found to have more than one cancer.

If this observation is true why is it that "only" 25 or 30 percent of the population dies from cancer? And why is it that many individuals live well into their eighties and nineties without developing any problems from the cancers that must be present in their bodies? The answer lies in the cancer concept of "promotional factors."

Cancer Promotion

Cancer experts say that on average most of us have several cells each day that mutate into a cancerous cell. The experts refer to this situation as "initiation," an apparently normal occurrence at any age.

They also tell us that the immune system is equipped to quickly detect and destroy these cancerous cells before they can multiply and enlarge into a colony of cells large enough to form a tumor.   Every now and then, however, a cancer cell develops the ability to elude detection and a tumor is born.   It is important for all of us to realize that in the early stages of tumor development the tumor is far too small for identification by any form of medical detection.

Often this growth is snuffed out as it becomes visible on the "radar screen" of the immune system. Or, it may just remain there in a state of limbo, contained, but not eliminated by the body's defenses. *It is this dormant, or latent, stage of cancer that virtually all of us over the age of 40 harbor.*

Again, these early stage cancers are not discovered because they are too small. You won't be aware of them. They produce no symptoms. They can't be detected by scans or x-rays. We only know they exist because of autopsy studies that use microscopic examination to find them.

As far as you or your doctor are concerned, there is no cancer present at all.

And as long as your immune system is operating effectively, and there are minimal "promotional factors" present, you will live a long, healthy life.

The term "promotional factors" refers to various influences and imbalances that favor the development of these small "latent" cancers into larger, clinically apparent malignancies - the kind that can kill you.

The precise mechanisms of these promotional factors on cancer development are not clearly understood. Hormonal imbalances certainly seem to play a promotional role. Stress, emotions, diet and nutrition, toxicity, and decreased energy production are other promotional factors.

Because of the decrease in energy production associated with the aging process, the immune system steadily loses efficiency. This decline, along with the other promotional factors I've just mentioned, permits further growth of cancer cells that would otherwise be mired in the latent, pre-clinical stage.

Ernest, 63, came to my clinic with a problem of uncontrolled blood sugar. He had been diagnosed with diabetes seven years previously. It turned out that the diabetes was secondary to a very rare condition created by cancer of the pancreas. Remember that the pancreas is the organ that produces insulin, the hormone that controls blood sugar.

Looking back on his medical history it became apparent that he had the cancer for at least eight years before its presence finally became apparent.

The case is typical of newly diagnosed cancers. By that I mean that the cancer is actually present and working in the body many years before clinical indications appear.

Many times physicians see patients who only a few weeks before were feeling fine but then suddenly have health complaints and symptoms of disease. As they investigate, the doctors discover bodies literally riddled with cancer. Often, such patients have passed annual physicals and blood tests that showed nothing abnormal.

Such experience tells us that without symptoms we are not yet sophisticated enough to recognize cancer in the formative pre-clinical stages. Once we have diagnostic tools to do so we would be in a more advantageous position to initiate therapy *before* the cancer reaches a malignant stage.

The Promise Of Early Detection Methods

Medical science is striving to develop reliable methods that would be able to determine the presence of "pre-cancer markers," that is, changes of naturally occurring substances in the blood that may indicate the promotion of a latent cancer into a malignancy.

I have already seen some promising tests and methods at work that give us an optimistic prospect for the future of cancer prevention.

One beneficiary of such budding technology has been my friend Dr. G, a pioneer in the field of alternative and anti-aging medicine. He looks to be about 50, has the energy and brain clarity of a 32-year-old, but is, in fact, 72.

Dr. G has been applying a variety of pre-cancer marker blood tests on himself "just to see." Two years ago one of these tests turned up some suspicious numbers. At first he thought the change was due to transient factors, but when the change persisted over the following twelve months, he became convinced that it was indicating that he had a latent cancer beginning to evolve into a malignancy.

The result didn't surprise him. His life for the past several years had been highly stressed. He had moved, set up a new clinic, started a new business venture, and typical for many of us in the medical profession, had too many irons in the fire.

Motivated by the results of the testing, he immediately set out to "clean up his act." His remedial efforts paid off. Within six months the blood test results began to reverse. One year later he tested completely normal.

Today, Dr. G is convinced that he cured himself of latent cancer that would have become malignant and potentially untreatable in three to five years. Such an assumption cannot, of course, be proven but I believe he is correct.

The case illustrates two important points:

1. It is highly likely that you and I already have latent cancers in the pre-clinical stage, and that under the influence of promotional factors such as stress, poor nutrition, smoking, and toxicity, these otherwise harmless cancers will evolve into a clinically detectable and potentially life threatening stage.

2. As the field of pre-cancer marker assessment further develops, *we will have the capability of detecting and treating cancers in their latent stage long before they become a life threatening malignancy.* By aggressively using safe, natural strategies to treat the

various promotional factors identified in each individual case, we should be able to prevent the development of most malignancies. Until the day that pre-cancer marker assessments become refined and widely available to doctors, it behooves us to recognize that the likelihood is great that we all harbor latent cancers in our bodies and to act accordingly. That means pursuing a prevention-oriented lifestyle that keeps cancer cells in confinement. Otherwise *you* are giving them the power to break out. It's like giving a convicted criminal the keys to the jailhouse. Following the recommendations in this book can help to keep these latent cancers in check.

Osteoporosis

Osteoporosis is a disease in which bones become fragile and more likely to break. If not prevented or if left untreated, bones indeed do break, typically in the hip, spine, and wrist. Because of the hormonal differences, four times more women are affected than men.

Americans have been brainwashed into thinking that a deficiency of calcium is the cause. The truth is that there are many factors causing osteoporosis but dietary calcium deficiency is not one of them. Osteoporosis is caused by excessive calcium loss, not deficient calcium intake.

That's a very important distinction to make, so I will repeat it. *The problem is excessive calcium loss, not deficient calcium intake.*

This distinction was very clearly emphasized by Neal Barnard, M.D., when he was commenting about Calcium Summit II. Calcium Summit II, held in January 2002, was a pseudo-scientific "health" conference sponsored by the National Dairy Council and the Milk Processor Education Program, as part of their ongoing effort to boost sagging milk sales.

According to Barnard, president of the Physicians Committee for Responsible Medicine, "Summit organizers say they brought together health professionals to look at what they claim is a calcium deficiency in youth, but studies show that increasing calcium intake does not increase bone strength."

Barnard goes on further to sate that, "A more useful public health measure would be to address *calcium loss.*"

Excessive calcium loss can be measured by monitoring the urine content of a substance called n-telopeptide. This is a much more useful way to assess bone health than bone density testing. It's inexpensive and only requires a urine specimen. Changes from therapy can be seen in less than two months. A distinct limitation of bone density testing is that the effects of therapy can't be fully evaluated for one to two years. That's a long time to wait to find out if a treatment is working!

N-telopeptide is a molecule that appears in the urine as a result of bone loss. The more bone loss that occurs, the greater the amount of n-telopeptide that appears in the urine. Successful anti-osteoporosis measures will demonstrate a decrease in urinary n-telopeptide levels in only 6-8 weeks. This makes it a very good way to immediately assess the effectiveness of your program.

Published studies clearly show that osteoporosis can be both prevented and treated by diet, exercise, vitamin D, sunlight, and hormone replacement. I have talked about all these issues in the book. Following these recommendations is all you need to keep your bones strong and youthful.

Is It Safe To Take Calcium Supplements?

Calcium is the most abundant mineral in your body. Ninety-eight percent of it is involved in building and maintaining strong bones. One percent goes to build and maintain your teeth. The remaining one percent is spread throughout the body and serves essential chemical roles in muscle contraction, blood clotting, and the transmission of nerve impulses. Normal bone health relies not just on calcium, but also on other minerals such as phosphorus, magnesium, silicon, strontium, and boron.

True calcium deficiency in this country is essentially non-existent. It doesn't turn up even in studies of inner city children, where researchers commonly find nutritionally deficient diets. The reason for this is that calcium is the only mineral with its own regulation system. When the level of dietary calcium falls, the body compensates by increasing calcium absorption from the intestines, and decreasing calcium loss from the kidneys. Calcium absorption is controlled by vitamin D, and calcium loss is controlled by parathyroid hormones. These systems work so well that a normal calcium balance will be maintained even with low calcium intake.

I believe that the indiscriminate supplementation of calcium to strengthen bones is not only useless but also dangerous. That's right, I said *dangerous*.

The food and supplement industries have achieved a major sales coup success by convincing women that they will develop osteoporosis unless they take calcium supplements. Actually, nothing could be further from the truth.

There is not a single well-controlled prospective study showing that calcium supplementation actually improves or even prevents osteoporosis. A prospective study just means that researchers follow a group of people for many years. Statistical studies that are not prospective are often subject to error.

Preventing osteoporosis with calcium supplements is a nice theory, and it seems to make sense, but it just doesn't pan out.

Instead of helping, supplementation can cause problems by putting an excess of calcium into the wrong parts of the body. Here are some of the worrisome potential dangers of excessive calcium consumption:

❏ Can Calcium Pills Cause Cancer?

What happens to someone taking supplementary calcium in spite of the fact that he or she does not have a deficiency? For starters, vitamin D production is suppressed. This leads to a deficiency of the vitamin.

In a 1999 study appearing in *Cancer Research*, a team of Harvard scientists cautioned against high calcium intake. They found that it increased the risk of advanced prostate cancer. Other studies have shown an equally disturbing relationship between increased calcium intake and the development of breast and colon cancer.

❏ Can Calcium Pills Cause Deficiencies?

Another problem with calcium supplementation relates to the absorption of other important nutrients. Specifically, calcium blocks the intestinal absorption sites for zinc and magnesium. By loading up on calcium you create a deficiency of these other factors. Many studies have confirmed that zinc and magnesium deficiencies are widespread.

❏ Can Calcium Pills Cause Heart Disease?

So what does the body do with all the excess calcium its getting that it doesn't need? The calcium certainly doesn't reach the bones, where you'd think it would go. Bone marker studies have clearly shown this. One common repository is the arteries, and yes, there's a connection here to calcified blood vessels, plaque, decreased circulation, and arterial obstruction.

Electron beam tomography represents a state-of-the-art diagnostic technique for coronary artery disease. Studies using this new technology quite clearly demonstrate that the chances of dying of a heart attack go up in direct proportion to the calcium content of the coronary arteries. This fact raises serious concern for the cardiovascular health of people consuming calcium pills.

❏ What Else?

All this is bad enough, but it's not the end of the story. In the body's attempt to deal with excess calcium intake, it channels the overload to the kidneys for urinary excretion. However, medical research informs us that this promotes kidney stones.

You'll also find calcium deposits in joints and tendons, thereby contributing to arthritis and tendonitis.

These facts certainly discourage me from recommending calcium supplements to patients. With what we know about how the body deals with calcium, it seems like wishful thinking to expect that supplementation will somehow magically restore bones without creating any of these undesirable effects.

If you examine the label of QuickStart™ you won't see calcium among the ingredients. Now you know why.

Depression

Depression often affects the elderly.

Why? The infirmities of aging, lost vigor, and lost loved ones give ample reason to be depressed, but these are not even the major reasons.

I believe that hormone deficiencies of estrogen, progesterone, thyroid, testosterone, and growth hormone are even more significant causes.

As an example, take the case of George, 64. He was reluctantly brought in by his wife of thirty-six years.

In front of him, she told me, "If you can't do something for him, I am going to lose my mind."

George had been a man of great passion and energy, but over the previous three years had become grumpy and complaining. Six months prior he had retired, and now he had no motivation and interest in life.

"At least he was bearable when he was working," his wife said. "But now that he's home all day, he drives me crazy with his complaints and demands."

George had tried counseling, but to no avail. He had no idea why he was so negative. It was completely uncharacteristic of him. Three different antidepressant medications had been tried and then stopped because of side effects and lack of efficacy.

Ordinarily, George enjoyed sex but admitted that, "If a naked super model walked in this room right now I wouldn't even look at her! I have absolutely no desire for sex."

During that first visit, George began to cry, and I saw in front of me a man who had given up, who felt utterly helpless and hopeless.

Testing revealed an abnormally low level of testosterone combined with an elevated level of estrogen. Both are common in men over sixty.

Bio-Energy Testing™ revealed a thyroid deficiency as well, even though his blood thyroid tests had been previously found to be within the "normal" range.

I prescribed natural thyroid and testosterone replacement, feeling that these would help elevate his depression and gusto. After three months, however, his condition had not improved even though his testosterone level was now normal.

Growth hormone replacement was an extremely expensive therapy at that time (1999), and for that reason I did not initially test him. I wanted to try other things first. But now the time had finally come to examine his growth hormone level. Not surprisingly it was quite low.

I then added growth hormone to his regimen.

After one month into this expanded program, George started to perk up.

When I reevaluated him in three months, his wife told me he was "almost back to his usual ornery self."

Ornery or not, George was thrilled.

No counseling. No drugs. Not even exercise in his case (he was extremely resistant to that suggestion!).

It was just a matter of giving his body the hormones that he so badly needed.

Just as an aside, George admitted to me that he had contemplated killing himself because he loved his wife too much to put her through the agony of living with him. He had never revealed his intention to me, or anyone else, because he planned to stage the suicide as an accident, so that his wife would collect his life insurance.

The case illustrates not only the powerful effect that hormones have on mood, but also the importance of prescribing *all* deficient hormones in order to optimize the therapeutic effectiveness. Since that time I have learned that testosterone replacement simply will not work in the presence of a growth hormone deficiency.

Unfortunately, many physicians are unaware of the astounding impact that hormones can have on the function of the brain, and especially on mood.

Diabetes

The latest statistics from the Centers for Disease Control indicate that nearly 16 million Americans - 6 percent of the population - have diabetes, the highest level ever recorded. Moreover, the incidence is increasing at the staggering rate of 798,000 new cases a year. That's equivalent to the population of Washington D.C., and about *six times* higher than the incidence in the early 1950s.

In my opinion, this development is a medical disgrace, a prime example of a distorted medical system that focuses almost entirely on treatment of symptoms while basically ignoring prevention. **Adult onset diabetes, a disease of modern living, is totally preventable.**

A recent survey revealed that only 8 percent of Americans regard diabetes as serious. Yet diabetes is deadly serious. It is the major cause of blindness, amputations, and kidney failure in adults, and a leading factor, as well, in nervous system disorders. Diabetic patients are also two to four times more likely to develop stroke and heart disease.

Adult onset diabetes is caused by high levels of blood glucose (sugar) resulting from flawed insulin secretion, insulin resistance, or both. As I discussed in the previous chapter, insulin is the hormone produced by the pancreas that controls blood sugar levels and moves sugar into the cells for use in energy production. In diabetes, insulin function is seriously compromised.

Adult onset diabetes is the most common form of the disease and develops slowly, usually among people over 45 who are overweight. However, health officials have started to see a disturbing increase in adult onset diabetes among children, a development that parallels the soaring rise of juvenile obesity.

The guidelines in this book will prevent diabetes.

One must do for diabetes prevention is exercise, which conditions the heart and blood vessels, lowers body fat, increases muscle weight, and increases cellular uptake of insulin and nutrients.

A 1998 study published in the *Journal of the American Medical Association* suggests that even mild exercise such as non-vigorous walking can "significantly" improve insulin sensitivity and reduce the risk of developing diabetes-related conditions.

A diet low in the high glycemic carbohydrates and regularly taking the ingredients and doses in QuickStart™ are also invaluable.

My Recommendations:

❑ See a prevention-oriented doctor. Don't wait until you have symptoms. A prevention specialist can put you on a program that reduces your risk of developing symptoms and illness. Regular checkups help to identify diseases earlier, making treatment more effective.

❑ Have an annual checkup. It is the best way to keep track of your health status and monitor progress as you strive to optimize your health. Is your preventive program really working to make you stronger, healthier, and functionally younger?

❑ Medicine is a rapidly changing field. Every year better diagnostic and therapeutic methods are being discovered, and it may be that your program can be improved or enhanced as a result of these developments. The annual checkup is a way to review and possibly update your program.

❑ As you grow older your needs will change, and so must your program.

❑ Assume you have pre-clinical cancers and act accordingly, taking better care of yourself and your immune system. Do this especially if you are going through a particularly stressful time in your life.

❑ Think of your fortieth birthday as a good point in life to see a preventive doctor for baseline studies. In fact, give yourself a birthday present in the form of a baseline evaluation. This evaluation should include Bio-Energy Testing™ and the other important tests mentioned throughout the book. The results of these studies on your health status at forty can be used as a base against which to compare your physiologic functions in later years as you age and embark on an anti-aging program.

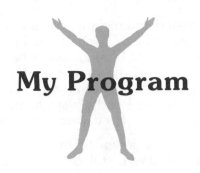

My Program

Seems no matter where I am talking, one question always comes up: "So what are your personal tests like, Doc, and what do you do to prevent aging?" I think the questioner is wondering if I really do everything I talk about. Well, the short answer is yes I do.

Chronologically, I am fifty-six years old. I feel and function every bit as good at this age as I did when I was in my twenties. And I feel a darned site *better* than I did only a few years ago. Here's my story.

Life In The Slow Lane

Up until the age of forty-six I raced bicycles and trained for ten to fifteen hours a week. I was extremely competitive despite the fact that I was a full time physician, a husband, and a father to four children. On most weekends, I would be out there competing in races that would often last three or four hours. This was my life for many years. I felt like a million bucks, and I could do things that most men my age could only dream about.

Then at the age of forty-six something happened that changed all that. I found myself not caring all that much about winning races, but caring more about spending time with my family and pursuing other activities.

So one day I quit racing.

I went from an intense exercise program of 2-3 hours a day to zero hours a day. I relished all my new found time. I enjoyed it so much that within six months I had gained 17 pounds.

In addition, I wasn't sleeping well. I was feeling unusually tired. I'd would ride up a mountain pass that I used to climb in just over 45 minutes, and now would not be able to get even half way up before succumbing to fatigue. I thought maybe I had developed hepatitis, an occupational hazard. Thankfully the tests were all negative. But other symptoms soon showed up that really got my attention.

I started to feel depressed and melancholic for absolutely no reason at all. Normally I had always been positive, optimistic, and enthusiastic about life to the extreme. Now I found myself being grumpy and negative. And I started to have all these aches. Where they came from I didn't know because I was not exercising or even doing much of anything strenuous. While racing I had always had a variety of aches and pains, but these were different. They were minor, but they were all over.

And then my sex life went down the drain. **Now at least I had a real reason to be depressed**. Of course there was always Viagra, but somehow this option was not all that comforting. I was a mess, but there was "nothing wrong" with me. My symptoms were non-specific, and all the blood tests were within normal limits.

As my 50th birthday grew closer I began to reflect on how my previous life of feeling and functioning in perfection was now being replaced by another life that I was not at all happy about. If this was my future, then things were really looking bleak.

And Then.....

And then one day in a flash of insight I finally figured it out. I was getting old. Or to put it more realistically, I was old! There was "nothing wrong" with me. I was just old. When I started comparing myself to patients of the same age I could see that they were going through many of these symptoms, too. But the reason they didn't perceive it as being a big problem, and had come to accept it as natural, was that they had deteriorated *gradually,* over ten to fifteen years. My fall was straight down, from feeling like a young man to feeling like an old man in only six months. Was this what women go through during the menopause?

Unbeknownst to me, my extreme exercise and fitness program had kept all the ravages of aging at bay, and it was only when I suddenly stopped that I began to feel my age. For fifteen years I had personally witnessed the incredible anti-aging power of exercise without ever fully realizing it. But I was realizing it now!

So armed with this new insight, I tested my hormone levels. Guess what? Not so hot. I was low on melatonin, growth hormone, DHEA, and testosterone. I started supplementing my program with melatonin, DHEA, and testosterone, and also started taking some growth hormone stimulating amino acids. In addition I began an exercise program.

This time the exercise was less fanatical than before, and was limited to a forty-five minute workout every weekday, and a two to three hour bike ride on the weekends. Within two months I was already starting to feel better. Eight months after I started making these changes I was back to feeling my old self again. It was as though I had just been given a new lease on life. I had experienced aging first hand and I did not like it one bit. I was glad to be rid of it, and I made a vow to do everything possible to make sure that I and my patients avoided it for as long as possible.

Fine Tuning

Several years later I learned about the testing technology that has now developed into Bio-Energy Testing™. When I tested myself I found that I was very low on thyroid, which at the time surprised me because my thyroid blood testing had always been in the normal range. In addition, I also learned that I was again testing low on growth hormone, this time in spite of the amino acid precursors I had been taking. So I started taking both thyroid and growth hormone.

I also discovered that my homocysteine level, my LDL cholesterol, and my lipo-protein (a) were all too high. The remainder of my tests were good.

I just had my Bio-Energy Testing™ repeated in April of 2002. My Fitness Factor was 110 indicating that my winter program of circuit training was working very well. My F.Q. was exactly 100 thus making my biological age forty years old. I hope to keep it at that level a long time.

My blood tests, blood pressure, arterial stiffness, heart and lung function, brain function, immune system function, strength, and balance are all optimal for a man in his thirties. My body fat is 12%.

Using the same information that I have spelled out in this book, I have created a personal program for myself that works just great. I've detailed it below. Remember that this is **my** program, geared to my individuality. You may very well require a more or less different program to achieve the same good results.

A Day In The Life of Frank Shallenberger

Diet: Low calorie, containing very little high glycemic carbohydrates. I eat very slowly and thoroughly enjoy my food. I only eat real food. No fast food...ever!

For breakfast I have two scoops of QuickStart™ blended with one tablespoon of flax oil, half an apple, a carrot, a half teaspoon of turmeric and two fresh ginger slices. I chase it with a cup of organic coffee.

For lunch I eat a salad with meat or cheese.

For supper I eat a combination of beans, veggies, meat, tofu, and salad. I usually have a glass of wine or a beer with supper. I don't normally eat dessert, but when I do, it's a real one. Not some form of packaged industrial waste!

Of course, sometimes I break the rules and misbehave, but by and large I stick with what I have described here.

Supplements: In addition to the QuickStart™ smoothie mentioned above, I take the following: 1000 milligrams of trimethylglycine and 5 milligrams of folic acid (to further lower my homocysteine level), 25 milligrams of DHEA, 3 grains of dessicated thyroid hormone, 1.5 milligrams of melatonin, 100 milligrams of CoQ10, 100 milligrams of lipoic acid, and 300 milligrams of niacin.

I also take 6 units of injectable human growth hormone in 10 divided doses every week, 3 months on and 1 month off.

Exercise: During the winter I circuit train for 35 minutes every other day, and I play tennis, weather permitting. In the summer, I ride my bike 60 -80 miles per week and slack off a little on the weights. I also backpack a good deal.

Miscellaneous: I log at least 8 hours of sleep, sunbathe whenever possible, and drink a quart of water every morning and evening. I use the breath meditation exercise every day, and have trained myself to breath abdominally even when exercising. I have a Bio-Energy Testing™ analysis performed once a year just to stay on top of any changes.

That's it. I know my program works well for me, because it keeps my Bio-Energy Testing™ numbers and all my other blood parameters looking optimal. And in addition, I love it because it's simple, easy, and sweet, just like me.

Putting It All Together

I've covered a huge amount of information in this book, including many recommendations. It's the same information and recommendations I give to my patients, and follow myself as I have just described.

I tell my patients that I would really like them to incorporate all the steps - all the secrets - into their everyday life. "Bursting with energy" isn't quite as simple (I wish it were!) as taking a single pill and voila....it's done.

It doesn't work that way. If I had that pill, I would be the richest man in the world.

The anti-aging and detoxification program I've outlined is an endeavor of a lifetime. The "secrets" need to become a routine part of daily life in order to live longer and healthier.

This is what I tell my patients. And then I very quickly add that I don't want them to feel overwhelmed. They shouldn't rush out and try to do everything at once. They should take my recommendations and carefully apply them in a sequential manner. Of course, with a patient, I can guide them personally, and prioritize the sequence according to their individual need and condition.

If you decide to pursue this comprehensive program, please give yourself time to adopt the changes. It is not in your interest, or in the interest of the program, to become pressured and stressed while trying to fashion a healthier lifestyle.

This is important. **Make it a point to find a Bio-Energy Testing™ facility and have your energy production capabilities thoroughly analyzed**. It is an absolutely amazing technology that is invaluable in many ways.

For best results, *all* the secrets in the program need to be addressed. That's because they work together.

As I said earlier in the book, how you eat affects how you exercise, how you exercise affects how you sleep, how you sleep affects how you view life, how you view life affects how you eat and exercise, etc.

209

I have laid out my recommendations - the "secrets" - in a sequence starting with the simplest steps. It's easy for instance, to start drinking more water. And getting more rest. And going out into the sunlight. Those are my first three "secrets."

Change is hard. Routine is easy. Once the changes I recommend become a part of your everyday life, they, too, can become routine and automatic.

But you can probably count on feeling some resistance at first, particularly if you are used to eating a certain way. And particularly if you are not used to exercising.

My supplement secret revolves around the use of QuickStart™.

The breathing recommendations can be applied easily, and when practiced over time, can also become an automatic part of your life.

Hormone replacement you can't do on your own. You'll need to find a prevention and anti-aging specialist. To do that contact either The American College for the Advancement of Medicine at 949-583-7666 (www.acam.org on the Internet) or The American Academy of Anti-Aging Medicine at 719-475-8775 (www.worldhealth.net). These organizations can provide referrals.

A word on weight loss. That's always a tough nut to crack. But the information I have provided you gives a new perspective on why you may be having a harder time than necessary to lose weight. Hopefully, this information will spark new inspiration. If you are very overweight, this is something you cannot put off. It is too critical to your energy, quality of life, and longevity.

Ideally, you should start adopting the recommendations as early as possible, and not wait until severe pain and debility make lifestyle changes that much more difficult to accomplish.

But at any age, and in any condition, when these changes are made, they will bring fresh energy into your life, and if you are ailing, they will improve, and perhaps even eliminate, your problem.

Just for the record, let me say that I follow my own preaching. I know first hand that it can be done, and that it is actually quite easy once you're used to it.

And I also know from my many patients that it works! When they follow the guidelines, they are literally "bursting with energy."

Many of my recommendations are designed to make you feel better immediately. But a lot of what I say has prevention in mind. These preventive measures are also very, very important for the long haul. Why would you want to feel better now, only to be sick later?

Medicine is changing as we speak. Soon, gone will be the days that seeing your doctor means that you are sick. Now, patients and physicians alike are finally getting the idea that seeing a doctor should be something you do *BEFORE* you are ill, in order to make sure that you don't become ill.

If your physician is already familiar with this concept, great! This is important because you will not be able to implement all the guidelines without an experienced physician working with you.

Get An Attitude!

Getting old is the perfect time to get a positive attitude. Enough cannot be said about the importance of attitude.

I haven't talked about it before, because I wanted to save it for last, but attitude can make or break any effort. And attitude governs how happily or unhappily you live life. And perhaps how long you live it as well.

Of course how long you live is really inconsequential compared to how well you live.

Did you hear the joke about the guy who goes in to see his doctor? After examining him and checking out all the tests, the doctor says: "You're going to have to stop drinking, skiing, smoking cigars, and chasing women."

"Will it make me live longer, Doc?" the patient asks.

"No, but I promise you that it will seem longer."

Joking aside, I can promise you that the sickness and pain and loss of function so commonly a part of the aging process will make your life seem longer as well, no matter what your age. For sure, that's not the kind of longevity I want for you. An aggressive anti-aging program following the recommendations in this book will insure that you don't experience that side of growing old.

> Growing old healthfully is just about the best thing that can happen to a person. It is a real gift. Make the most of it.

Don't pay any attention to all the negative cultural messages implying that you're over the hill. Sure, when you were younger you could do things twice as fast, but you enjoyed them only half as much!

Don't Yield To aging.

The senior years represent the only time in our lives when we are wise enough to really enjoy all that life has to offer.

The key is that while you grow old chronologically you don't have to keep pace biologically. You can be younger-feeling while you are getting older. That's what "bursting with energy" is all about.

Nor do you have to grow old psychologically. Think young! Ask yourself, "Is there anything I would do now if I were only younger?"

Whatever the answer is, do it!

This is your life. Live it to the fullest until it ends.

Now is a great time to rid yourself of negative attitudes and assumptions that get in the way.

I don't have any great words of wisdom here, except to remind you that all things are possible when we open up our hearts and let love in. Love is the ultimate vitamin. If you are not in love with someone or something, it is important to work on this. Ask yourself what it is that you love. Cultivate and value connections with people, animals, plants, mountains, lakes, bicycles, your car, whatever...

Appreciate all your good qualities, and work on developing more. Accept full responsibility for every aspect of your life. For what has gone wrong, and for what has gone right. This is what free will is all about, and the realization of this is the source of all your power, including the power to get well and stay well.

The four most important aspects of life are relationships, money, work, and health. All require some work. They are *never* dialed in. They constantly change, and must be continuously re-examined.

Get some professional counseling if you need it. There is no one who can't benefit from counseling every now and then.

Happiness is not a goal. It's a path. And so is contentment in who you are, and how you live your life. Don't compare yourself to others. It is a waste of valuable time. There will always be someone who is better, and someone who is worse, so what's the point**?**

Whenever possible, sing, dance, pray, rejoice, and laugh...especially at yourself.

Be forgiving with yourself. If you don't forgive yourself, you won't be able to forgive others.

Lastly, don't be afraid to try on new attitudes. It's OK to make mistakes at any age. Mistakes are how we learn. They are lessons, and you are going to get a lot of lessons in your life. If you don't make mistakes and learn from them, you don't grow. Imagine how smart you're going to be after an entire lifetime of mistakes.

Good Luck.

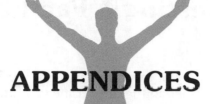

APPENDICES

Appendix A
How To Find A Bio-Energy Testing™ Facility

As of the printing of this book, Bio-Energy Testing™ centers are being established in the San Francisco Bay Area and in Southern California. Other centers will soon be established throughout the United States. For more information please call toll free 1-866-376-0610, or go to www.bursting-with-energy.com on the Internet.

Appendix B
QuickStart™ Ingredients

D r. Shallenberger is licensed both as a Medical Doctor and a Homeopathic Medical Doctor, and has been practicing nutritional and preventive medicine since 1978. During that time he has analyzed the biochemical and nutritional needs of literally thousands of patients. He discovered that there were certain nutrients and herbs which he found all his patients were in need of, and so he decided to put all these ingredients in their full doses in one easy to take product, "Dr. Shallenberger's Super Immune QuickStart™.

While it is in no way a substitution for a healthy diet, the spectrum and doses in this mixture reflect the current state of the art in nutritional supplementation and detoxification. *When used in conjunction with flax oil and a three week detoxification program of exercise and abstention from coffee, alcohol, sweets, flour, and milk, Dr. S's QuickStart™ formula prevents and often cures many problems and disorders without any other needed intervention.*

Pills vs. Food

Dr. Shallenberger developed this unique green drink more than 15 years ago, and since then its popularity has spread across the country simply by word of mouth. It is the only "one stop" nutritional product available which, when prepared as directed, provides all the supplementary nutrition, detoxification, and immune enhancement that most people will ever need, in an easy and affordable "power breakfast" smoothie.

There are four basic reasons for these advantages:

1. Much of the vitamin content of commercial supplements in tablet and capsule form is ruined in the manufacturing process.

2. Many individuals are not able to adequately break down tablets and capsules. Thus, much of the contents are not absorbed. All the nutrients in QuickStart™ are prepared as a fine powder. The special processing protects nutrient values and enhances absorption potential, even for those with less than perfect digestive systems.

3. It would require more than 60 horse pills (I mean big pills) in order to equal the same amount of nutrients found in a routine dosage of QuickStart™. Very few people will take that many capsules for very long.

4. Dr. Shallenberger has carefully formulated this product so that each vitamin, mineral, and herb is present in the exact form that he has found to be the most clinically effective.

Our Immune Systems Under Siege

What causes one person to catch a flu and another to avoid it? Why does one person develop an immune related disease while another living in the same environment doesn't? Why do some people have allergies? Why do serious outbreaks of infectious diseases leave some individuals untouched? The answers of course lie within our immune systems. *From viruses never before discovered to antibiotic resistant bacteria, our immune systems are being challenged in ways we have never seen before*. These days we really need to have the most supercharged immune systems imaginable. Through diet, adequate rest, and the special nutrients in Dr. S's formula you will harness your body's ability to do the job that nature intended: combat and prevent disease.

The Ultimate Prescription

Over the years, Dr. Shallenberger's patients have reported a noticeable improvement in many different kinds of conditions, despite the fact that frequently QuickStart™ was all they were taking. This is because QuickStart™ works on such basic, fundamental levels, providing antioxidant protection and nutritional insurance, while at the same time enhancing immunity, alkalinizing tissues, improving brain function, improving circulation, and detoxifying the liver and intestinal tract. *Because it is so low in carbohydrate, while increasing metabolism and stabilizing appetite, it is the perfect supplement for any weight control program*. Try it for three months and you won't believe how good you feel.

As per federal guidelines, we need to inform you that these statements have not been evaluated by the FDA. This product is not intended to diagnose, treat, or cure any disease. If you are sick please consult a physician.

2 Scoops QuickStart™ Contain:

30,000 IU beta Carotene

10,000 IU Vit A

2,000 mg Vit C

400 IU Vit E (d-alpha)

1000 mg Hesperidin Bioflav Complex

120 mg Ginkgo Biloba Extract

600 mg Magnesium (citrate)

10 mg Manganese (amino acid chelate)

300 mg Potassium (citrate)

200 mcgm Selenium (selenate)

1200 mcgm Chromium (picolinate)

16 mg Zinc (picolinate)

2 mg Copper (amino acid chelate)

100 mg B1

50 mg B2

100 mg Niacin

300 mg Pantothenic Acid

100 mg B6

1000 mcgm B12

1000 mcgm Folic Acid

500 mcgm Biotin

300 mg Astragalus Extract

6 grams Spirolina Pacifica

750 mg L-Glutamine

100 mg n-Acetyl Cysteine

320 mg Saw Palmetto

5 grams psyllium husks

5 grams stabilized rice bran

5 grams soy protein isolate

5 grams whey protein (undenatured)

Appendix C
How to Order QuickStart™

QuickStart™ can be ordered by calling the toll-free number 1-866-377-0610. As an alternative it can also be ordered onlin at www.bursting-with-energy.com.

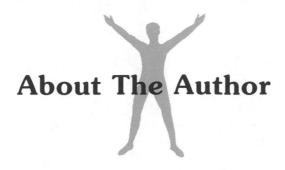

About The Author

Frank Shallenberger, M.D., has devoted his professional career to understanding the fundamentals of what keeps us well. To this end, he has used an approach in his medical practice for more than twenty years that integrates the best of alternative medicine with the best of conventional medicine.

He is a pioneer in the clinical application of oxidative medicine, a new discipline that emphasizes the profound importance of oxygen and energy production in health and longevity. Using a revolutionary technology known as Bio-Energy Testing™ he is able to measure the energy production of patients, and improve it to more youthful levels.

Shallenberger is the founder and medical director of The Nevada Center of Alternative and Anti-Aging Medicine in Carson City, Nevada, a facility that attracts patients from all over the country. He is board certified in Anti-Aging Medicine, and has served as a Clinical Instructor in Family Medicine at the University of California School of Medicine in Davis. In 2001 he was a keynote speaker at the First International Learning Conference on Anti-Aging Medicine in Monte Carlo, a global gathering of health professionals interested in applying anti-aging strategies.

Shallenberger's family includes wife, four children, two grandchildren, a horse, and five chickens. He is an avid backpacker and cyclist. He has won numerous cycling events, and garnered silver medals in the Nevada State Mountain Bike Championship Series and the Northern California Time Trials.

He aims to keep himself and his patients young and energetic for a long time.